Understanding Medical Statistics

Leonard A. Goldstone,
B.A.(Econ.), M.Sc., F.S.S.

Head of School of Health Studies,
Newcastle upon Tyne Polytechnic, UK

William Heinemann Medical Books Limited
London

William Heinemann Medical Books Limited
23 Bedford Square
London WC1B 3HH

ISBN 0-433-12402-4

First published 1983
Reprinted 1985

Printed and bound in Great Britain by
the Alden Press, Oxford

Foreword

Books on medical statistics are almost too numerous, but good ones are rare—because few people have the gift of exposition where statistical ideas are concerned. Something like the truth, from a strictly mathematical point of view, has to be set in a clinical context which looks real, and interesting. When I was a medical student in Liverpool Lord Cohen of Birkenhead, a great teacher who was our Professor of Medicine, used to tell the story of a very ill man who consulted a surgeon. He was told that he needed a desperate operation but would certainly be all right: 'How can you be so sure?' he asked; and the surgeon confidently replied, 'The mortality rate for this operation is 90%; I have done nine cases so far and they have all died!' This is the art of conveying a big lesson through a little story; a serious message through a twist of humour. It shows the same teacher's insight as that of the man who first pointed out that half the people in this country are below average IQ; it makes the student think but it helps him to do it, and enjoy it.

I have tried to teach medical statistics, without knowing any (which some people might think is the best way) and I have made my own attempt at writing an explanatory chapter on the subject, in a book on analgesic drugs. I have sought help from a number of people, over the years, in arranging courses on medical statistics. I am well able to appreciate Leonard Goldstone's qualities as the sort of teacher we are all looking for, and I think these qualities radiate through the text of his book.

The course that Leonard refers to, in which we both took part, was interesting in that the participants came from all levels of medical practice, including newly qualified doctors, consultants and a professor. This gave us no problems; indeed, it showed that there are great opportunities for bringing together people at various stages of their careers. The real difficulties in helping doctors with medical statistics are, first, the very wide differences in requirement, for instance between psychiatrists, epidemiologists and radiotherapists; and second, the even wider differences in educational groundwork at school level, between most British doctors and those who have come from other countries. No single course can solve everyone's problems and neither can any single book; it has to be assumed that a certain starting point can be attained, and then the emphasis, in a general book, must be on setting out the principles and the scope of the subject. I feel that this book makes sensible assumptions, and gives excellent coverage in these respects. It will make you think, it will make you smile; it will perhaps make you question, and if it arouses your interest in probability as well as the routine of significance testing, I shall not be surprised.

Professor J. Parkhouse,
Postgraduate Dean and
Director of the Regional
Postgraduate Institute,
Regional Postgraduate Institute
for Medicine and Dentistry,
University of Newcastle upon Tyne,
UK

Preface

This book is deliberately very concise, keeping to principles rather than detail. The exposition is verbal and arithmetic, rather than algebraic. The emphasis is on intuitive understanding rather than on proof or mechanical aspects of calculations, although some calculations are illustrated where appropriate. The examples are simplified and go from the particular to the general, rather than the reverse, which is more usual. Great care has been taken over the decisions about what to omit. The subject has been carefully stripped of its frills, of proofs, of statistical symbols which would not further the doctor's understanding, of detail of techniques which might well in practice be left to a computer or calculator, and of particular methods which are not essential during the acquisition of a basic understanding.

There remain the essentials of the subject—the bits every doctor should understand. These essential concepts are all included in a way which is not jargon-based and not symbol-bound. Together with the traditional statistical topics, there is a discussion on computers, and some management related material.

Whilst the book has been written for, and as a consequence of working with, doctors, it contains a great deal of material of interest and relevance to medical students, health visitors, district nurses, hospital nurses, physiotherapists and occupational therapists.

Leonard A. Goldstone

Contents

Acknowledgements

I should like to acknowledge my gratitude to Professor James Parkhouse of the University of Newcastle who, by hiring me almost unseen many years ago to run some three-day courses on 'Statistics for Anaesthetists' launched my career into a new direction. I am also indebted to the many medical researchers whom I subsequently met who asked for statistical assistance and thus enriched my own knowledge of techniques and applications.

I have given many courses on statistics to doctors, in the context of health management courses with a mixed professional group, and frequently to young doctors working towards their Primary Fellowship examinations. This book originates in some lecture notes for the latter group, which were extremely popular and in high demand despite their being in existence already several excellent texts on medical statistics. The notes grew to a book whilst the author fought off attempts to include every statistical technique that has ever appeared in a journal. I am grateful to all the doctors who argued with me as to which techniques I should include. I have tried to strike a balance between over-inclusion and over-omission. I hope the book is short and clear enough to make statistics interesting, relevant and readable.

1

Introduction

'He who accepts statistics indiscriminately, will often be duped unnecessarily. But he who distrusts statistics indiscriminately will often be ignorant unnecessarily.'

W.A. Wallis and H.V. Roberts, in *Nature of Statistics*, The Free Press, New York, 1965

'. . . an apparently objective 'fact' transmitted as a number may have precision but total inaccuracy, whilst an apparently subjective description may be vague, but accurate and communicative of the true situation.'

S.J. Kilpatrick, in *Statistical Principles in Health Care Information*, University Park Press, Baltimore, 1977

The practice of medicine is closely bound up with probability and statistics.

Probability in its traditional definition relates the observed frequency of an event to the number of times it might have occurred. For example, if you treat an illness in 100 patients and have three 'successes', then you might speculate about the next patient that there is a 3% or 0·03 probability of success.

There is also a concept of probability for situations where we have no previous experience. For example, just before the first heart transplant the surgical team must have had some degree of faith that the outcome would be favourable. They may well have said that they expected a 50:50 chance of success. If this is so we can put this another way by saying they envisaged that the probability of success was 50%, or 0·5, even though they had no previous experience to go on.

This type of probability is essentially subjective, and obviously more controversial than the relative frequency definition. To use subjective probability requires a re-definition such as 'a measure (between 0 and 1) of the legitimate intensity of belief that an event or outcome will occur'. Probability can thus be revised as new knowledge becomes available. Thus, whilst 0·03 is the probability of success for an unseen patient in our earlier example, once the patient presents himself for examination, the doctor may feel that he has a higher or lower probability than 0·03. Probability is important in medical decision making and implicitly underlies diagnosis, prognosis and treatments.

The word 'statistics' has two principal meanings. If we consider a collection of numerical facts describing people or a system, each fact or piece of information is a 'statistic', and collectively the plural is 'statistics'. Thus, your height is a statistic—and so is mine. Together they are 'statistics', and if we extend our coverage, for example, to the population of the United Kingdom we can collect about 56 million of these 'height' statistics. We can also note other statistics such as weight, blood pressure, and so on, and build up, statistically, a medical description of our population, and going on from here we could begin to assemble the information into meaningful summaries and diagrams. We may choose samples, attempt to make inferences and test hypotheses and assess whether relationships exist. The art and science of assembly, classification, inference, hypotheses testing and so on is referred to as 'statistics', a singular noun.

Both plural and singular use of statistics are essential to doctors whose interests range from general practice through to specialisation and associated biological and other scientific work, community medical care and health service management.

One of the main goals of medical undergraduate education is to produce doctors who are efficient at diagnosis, prognosis, and prescription and management of treatment. Each of these has a statistical basis: 'statistics' is thus not 'external' to medicine, but rather integral to its main functions.

For example, diagnosis relies on classification, which is ultimately a statistical idea. A diagnostic group is deemed to exist when a particular group of symptoms and manifestations occurs together more frequently than would happen by chance, and when the combination appears to have relevance for prognosis or treatment, and can be understood or explained in the context of current medical knowledge. Once 'diagnoses' are available, then individuals need to be matched to the appropriate diagnosis. The doctor has to make this decision on the basis of information about a unique patient who may not have all the relevant symptoms, or more than those appropriate to a particular diagnosis. Consequently, the decision on a particular patient's diagnosis is an exercise in applied probability.

Prognosis similarly is essentially probabilistic and statistical, deriving from observations and records on previous similar cases. The doctor needs to know the proportion of comparable sufferers of the disease in question who have survived for specific periods, or have experienced particular outcomes.

Choice of treatment also depends on statistical information. In the light of previous experience of the treatment—again statistical records—a specific treatment can be prescribed. The chosen regime is the one which maximises the probability of success.

From now on, when we use the word 'statistics' to mean the collection of techniques available for data analysis, we will for convenience include probability within this set.

Statistics in recent years have become more important in medicine, partly because of demands for properly conducted trials of new treatments, the results of which can only be interpreted using statistical knowledge, and partly because of the availability of inexpensive calculators and the advent of 'canned' statistical programs on more and more widely available computers. The ease with which results can be analysed by many techniques means that the literature of medicine abounds with statistical tests and terminology. The doctors involved in the research process which leads to the statistics do not need to be familiar with every statistical and mathematical detail of the techniques they use. But, it is extremely dangerous not to understand the fundamental ideas and assumptions underlying the techniques. Those who subsequently read and act on the reported results must also be able to evaluate the research and understand its statistical limitations. This book is concerned with basic concepts which must form part of the stock-in-trade of every doctor who must make decisions based on the use of statistics.

Objections and Difficulties

Antipathy towards statistics acts as a barrier to the use and acceptance of statistical results. This barrier is partly due to the feeling that people are best treated individually as people, rather than statistics. This is of course a view fully justified at the 'bedside' level, but one which cannot be maintained at a more macro level where we may be planning for services, or carrying out trials. At the 'higher' level we need to speak in general overall terms about the population, and we can only do this in terms of statistics. A general result may be derived from statistical analysis, namely that policy A or treatment B is appropriate for the disease C with symptoms D, E and F. The general result does not conflict with the possible judgement by a doctor that, in view of individual circumstances and factors for patient X, some alternative regime is to be employed. It is important to accept that statistics do not make medical judgements or prescribe. The results of statistical analysis are one of the inputs in a doctor's decision making, not a substitute for individual diagnosis, interpretation and policy.

Another barrier to the use of statistics is the difficulty involved in learning about statistical methods. Many of the textbooks are too difficult and complex for the non-mathematician to read. Most resort to the use of symbols at the earliest opportunity, and use them as an abbreviation. Whilst symbolic notation is a boon for the mathematician, and essential for development of theory, it becomes an extra hurdle for the non-statistician to master before he can come to grips with the statistical concepts. The present volume differs from tradition by minimising, and almost excluding, the use of symbols, minimising the inclusion of algebra, and wherever possible using words and an intuitive explanation. It is frequently asserted that 'you can prove anything with statistics', and that 'there are lies, damned lies, and statistics'. There is no doubt that those, who for various reasons are intellectually dishonest can misuse statistics. When nine out of ten women prefer brand X, it is entirely reasonable for the advertiser to state this. We need to know who asked the question, and how it was phrased. We also need to know the sample size and how it was chosen, and we need an estimate of the error associated with 'nine out of ten' when it is transferred from the sample to the population. In short, much of the misuse of statistics which causes—quite rightly—scepticism comes from failure to supply necessary associated information, or from highly selective reporting, or from deliberately contrived presentation, such as graphs where the scales are chosen to emphasise a particular feature.

Normal and Variation

A great deal of statistical analysis is concerned with variation. Variation in biological measurements is quite usual. It would be quite astonishing if all men were the same height or weight or had the same haemoglobin levels. Doctors need a way of saying when a measurement which differs from average is sufficiently different to be abnormal or 'pathological'. Every variable has a distribution from the lowest value to its highest value, usually with some clustering around the average. Doctors need an understanding of the nature and density within such distributions to help with decisions on what is normal or non-pathological. In particular a measure of the variation in the population of comparable patients is essential background information to be set against departure from the average for any individual. Problems such as the classification of groups of like members, comparison of treatments, and the ascription of cause begin with a measurement of variation. When we identify and understand the factors which generate variation, then the first steps to control are being taken and meaningful assessments of treatments, or factors, etc., which are associated with the variation, can begin. For example, in a situation where there are sound theoretical reasons for supposing that a measure, such as IQ, depends on two or more joint explanatory variables, such as heredity and environment, then to resolve the argument as to which is more important we would first need to measure the variation in IQ to be explained in a suitable sample, and then assess how much of the variation is due to variation in heredity, and how much to environment.

Both medical researcher and doctor–user need a thorough understanding of variation, its measures, and the reliability of methods of estimating its causes to, respectively, put the best into and get the most out of medical literature whilst understanding the limitations of the methods in use.

Conclusions

Medicine, medical research and medical journals abound with statistical tests and analysis. Not all are entirely correctly concluded and interpreted. For a realistic appraisal of the value and methodology in the work, the medical student, practising doctor, or researcher must understand the fundamental principles of statistics.

This book concentrates on fundamentals. It is not a cookbook of formulae, nor a detailed comprehensive statistical tome. It provides an understanding without the clutter of mathematical symbols. In note form it has had great success in the Department of Postgraduate Medical Education at Manchester University, from whose students the request for copies stimulated expansion and publication.

The book is deliberately concise. Statistics is a vast area of theory and practice. Accordingly, the book is highly selective and concentrates on those topics which are both fundamental and of widest use.

Some of the most important topics in medical statistics are the presentation, description and summarising of numerical information; probability; drawing inferences from and testing hypotheses using sample information; the analysis of inter-relationships; clinical trials and experimental design; analysis of vital statistics; calculations relevant to resource utilisation; and the statistical use of computers. The following chapters treat the basic features of each topic in an essentially verbal and intuitive manner.

Probability, in the context of this book, began 'life' as Chapter 5. I am grateful to readers and reviewers who suggested that because they 'sailed' through the manuscript prior to Chapter 5, and came to an abrupt intellectual halt on the probability material, I should remove the chapter on probability and insert it as an appendix. Because probability is so important to statistics I have endeavoured to compensate for its removal to the appendices (see Appendix 2) by introducing it as a usable concept from page 1 of the Introduction, mentioning it as appropriate and as often as possible thereafter, to ensure familiarity without hampering readability.

2

Diagrams and Charts

In descriptive statistics we make use of a number of simple diagrams to convey the magnitudes of numbers in a manner which a reader will find easy to understand and assimilate. If a diagram is complex, covering many variables, it may be better either to construct an efficient and neat tabulation or to present a short series of simple diagrams. It is often better to present less information clearly than to construct one composite diagram which contains everything, but which is very difficult for the reader to disentangle.

The most common devices for presentation are the graph, the bar chart, the pie chart, the pictogram, and the histogram. Each of these has a number of variants, but we refer here to basic examples, pointing out features which contribute to good style.

The Bar Chart

The bar chart can be used to chart the progress of a variable through time, or it can compare the level of the variable at several locations. The area of the bar is proportional so the magnitude being represented. Usually all the bars are the same width, so the height is proportional to the magnitude.

The 'time' use is much the same as if we were using a simple graph, but the uniqueness of each month is emphasised by an individual bar drawn for that month. In a simple graph the points representing each month are joined up and suggestions of trend are easier to make. Figures 1(a) and 1(b) show, respectively, a simple graph and a bar chart presentation of the percentage of surgical wound infections in all operations in a general hospital

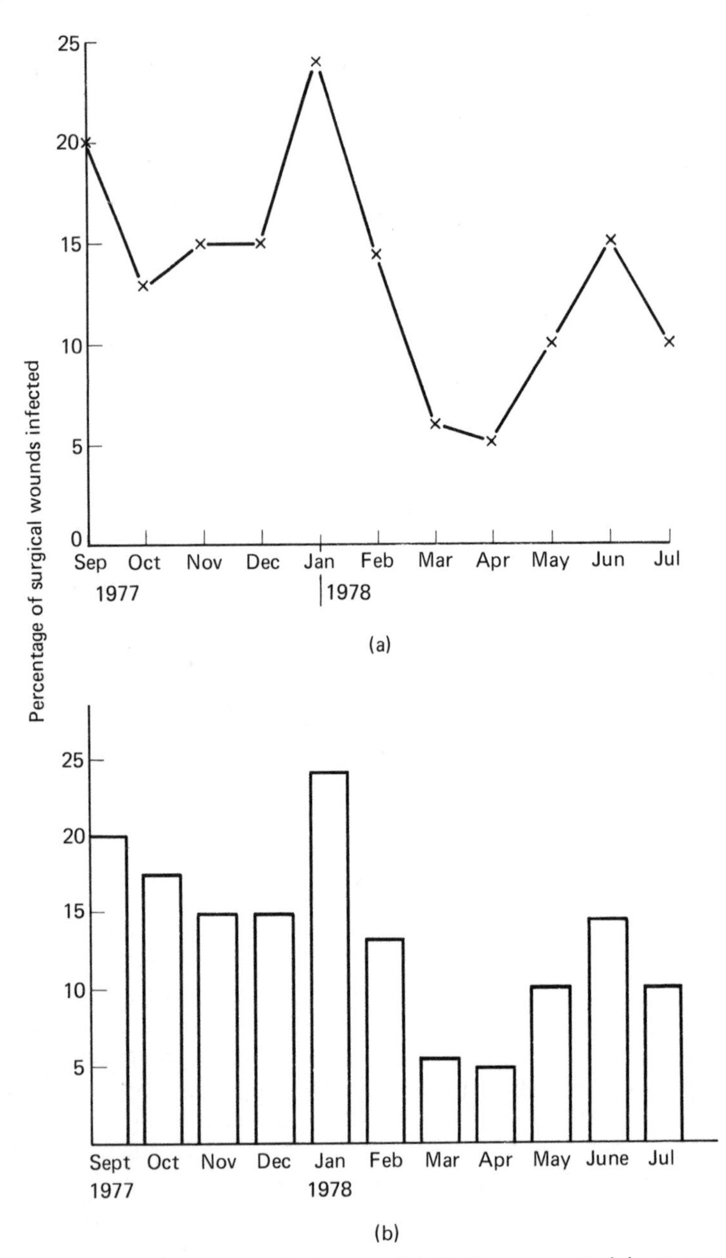

Fig. 1. Percentage of surgical wound infections reported in a general hospital.

for an 11-month period. For the bar chart the gap between bars should differ from the width of the bars to facilitate interpretation. Often, absence of shading or cross-hatching is a positive advantage. For the reader the diagram can be just an informative, and for the presenter considerable time may be saved. Cross-hatching can also be quite confusing and be optically somewhat disturbing.

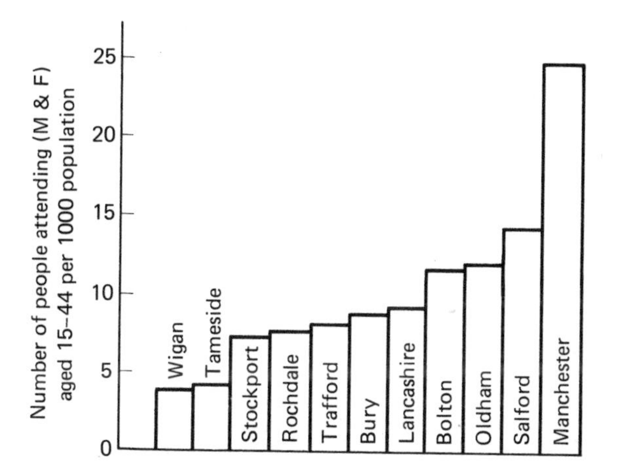

Fig. 2. Rank-order bar chart showing the variation over areas in attendances at sexually transmitted disease clinics (1975).

Figure 2 shows the bar chart in use for comparison of attendances at clinics in different towns. Here there is no horizontal scale, merely the names of the towns. Putting the bars in rank order is a useful feature. A useful variant of the bar chart is the component bar chart illustrated in Figs. 3 and 4 and the '100%' component bar chart in Fig. 5. Here we see the total built up from its components. As before, the gaps between should differ from the bar widths, and where a comparison, as opposed to a time study is being made, a rank order approach may be beneficial. It is also advantageous to keep to a maximum of four components in each bar, and to put the largest at the bottom, with decreasing rank order towards the top. To mix up the ranks within bars is to risk sandwiching the smaller sections and apparently reducing their importance. Obviously the same order should obtain in each bar, and so where a rank order change is present in the data the

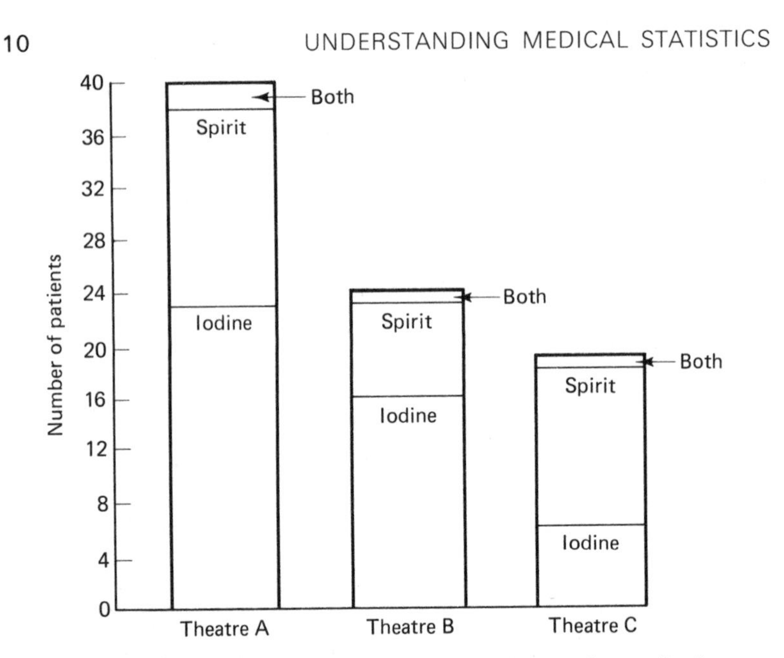

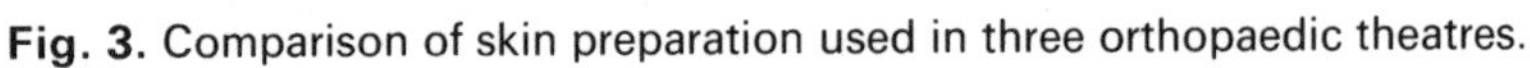

Fig. 3. Comparison of skin preparation used in three orthopaedic theatres.

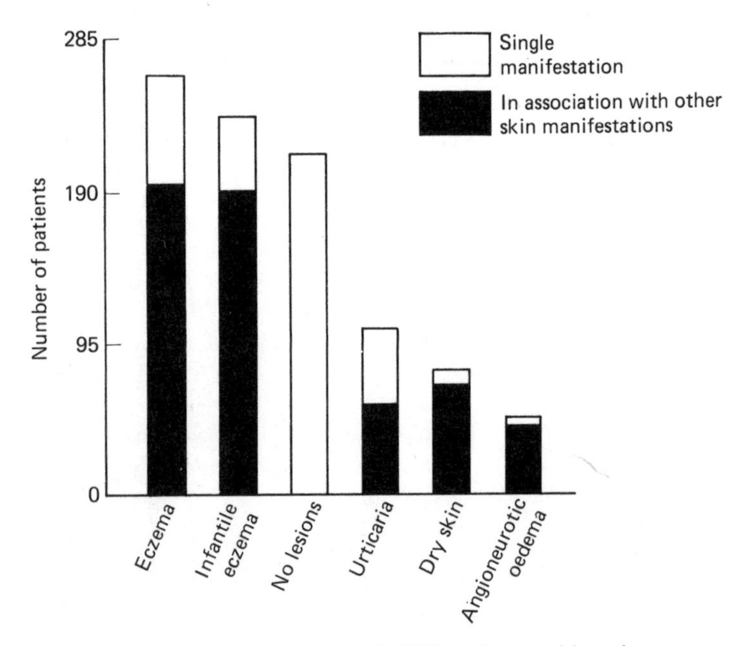

Fig. 4. Skin manifestations in 952 children with asthma.

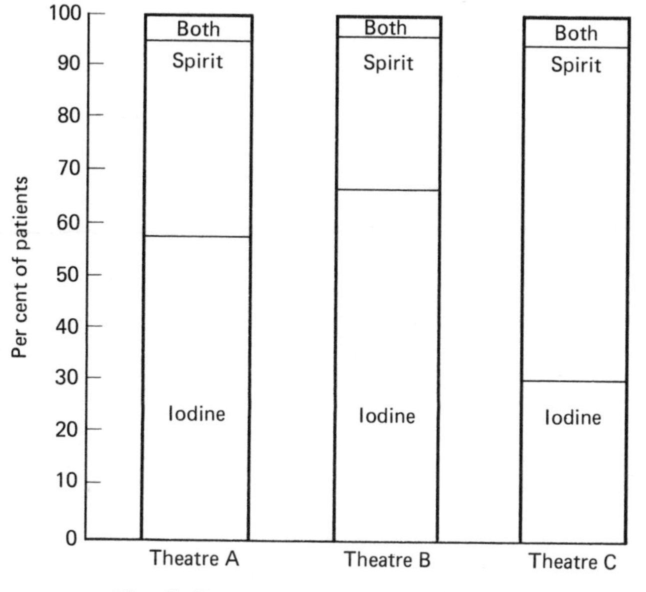

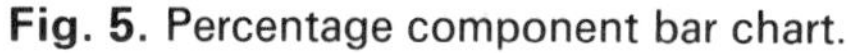
Fig. 5. Percentage component bar chart.

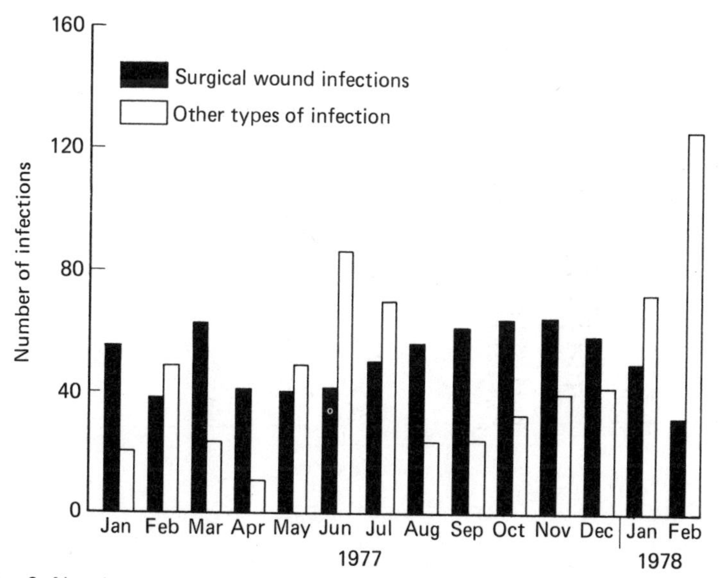

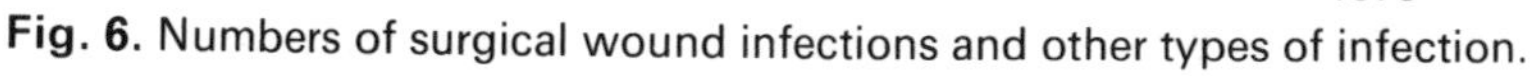
Fig. 6. Numbers of surgical wound infections and other types of infection.

component which is usually largest should be at the base, that which is usually second largest above it, and so on.

Cross-hatching, especially with parallel lines in opposing directions, should be minimal, and solid shading is preferable if any is to be done at all. Frequently it is possible to save time and convey the information just as efficiently by writing the names or identifiers of the components into them, without the need for varying shading.

If shading is to be used, the large components at the base should be darker, and the shading should reduce in intensity for smaller components above.

An alternative is the component bar chart shown in Fig. 6 where totals are not present. Components are more easily compared with each other and themselves over time, or between locations. Obviously the totals, if required, can be the subject of a separate presentation. (The scale required for effective display of the components may not always permit the total to be included in the same diagram as the components.)

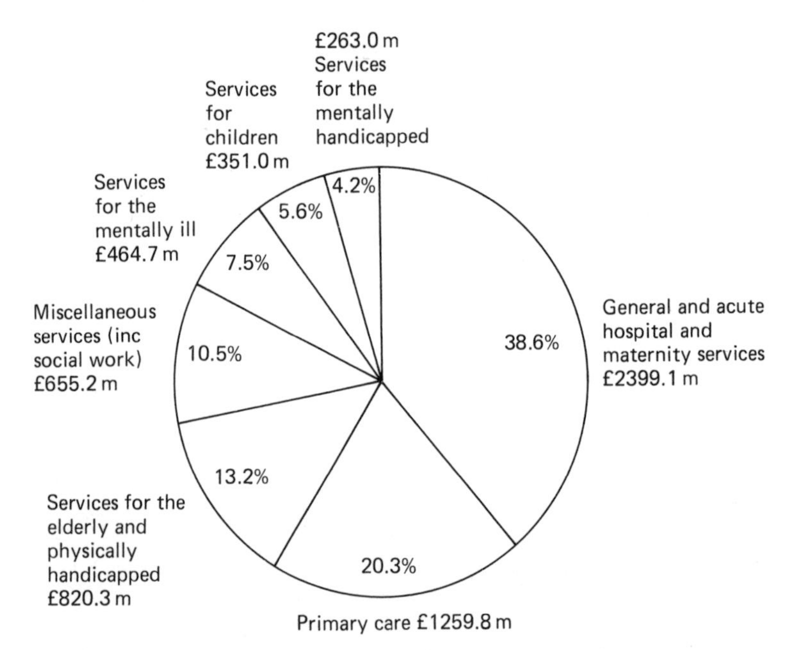

Fig. 7. A pie diagram for National Health Service and Personal Social Services Current Expenditure, England 1977–78 (1978 prices). Source: Report of the Royal Commission on the National Health Service. (Cmnd 7615, 1979, Table E1.)

The pie diagram shows the split of a total into its constituent parts. The 360° angle at the centre is apportioned to each item in the total in proportion to importance. The most effective pie diagrams have no more than five or six sectors, with the largest starting at the vertical (12 o'clock) and proceeding clockwise, followed in rank order by the other sectors. If shading and cross-hatching is omitted then full identification and some statistical detail can be written into each sector (Fig. 7).

The pictogram is primarily used for presentation to laymen. It is possible to represent magnitudes by simplified pictures. Thus, for example, the number of doctors per 1000 people can be illustrated using multiples of dry transfers of pictures of men. When there are fractions of a doctor involved, the possibilities as to which part of the anatomy is used presents a real problem.

Using magnified pictures of the same entity is even more open to misinterpretation. Thus, if we wished to represent a situation where the incidence of a disease is twice as great in one place as another, then to use a picture of a man who is twice as tall is misleading because he will be twice as wide (and, though this may not be illustrated, twice as deep). Thus, the apparent information is that incidence is up by a factor of 4 (or 8 in the case of a diagram with a three-dimensional aspect).

The histogram is a particular type of bar chart which differs from the two we have so far considered. We have either had a horizontal time scale or a series of 'labels' on the horizontal axis, when bar charts have been drawn. In the case of the histogram, the horizontal scale is a measure of the magnitude of some variable in which we are interested. Subdivisions of the scale into classes is made by the individual constructing the histogram, and the vertical scale shows the frequency of occurrence of items or entities within those classes. The following chapter presents more detail on the histogram.

Conclusions

Diagrams, if they are to be effective, need to be simple in design, and carefully chosen to illustrate the point being made. A few simple diagrams usually are preferable to one complex picture, and those diagrams drawn need to follow some of the rules for good style described in this chapter.

3

The Mean, Other Averages, and the Histogram

Introduction

Medical data frequently consists of a large batch of numbers, often measurements of a group of patients. Table 1 contains 70 measurements of birthweight of all the premature babies born in a particular unit at hospital X in 1980. Just by looking at the weights in the table it is obvious that considerable variation is present in the weights, and that taking a simple average and using this to characterise the group ignores the important dimension of variation.

Many of the medical and nursing decision policies and problems stem from the variability from baby to baby, and so when we ask 'on average what birthweights are we dealing with in the premature unit?' we should also require to know 'how much variation is present?'. To present all 70 members in a table certainly indicates the variation, but will be unhelpful to the reader who cannot absorb a mass of numerical information immediately. In cases of greater numbers of observations this difficulty is exacerbated. In particular, if we wished to make comparisons with another group this is not feasible on the basis of a comparison of the raw data in tabular form such as in Table 1. The problem of measuring 'average' values and 'levels of variability' will be resolved by calculating a few simple summary statistics, which then facilitate comparison with other groups.

Mean, Median and Mode

Any summary of the 'raw' data in Table 1 should contain a 'typical' 'central', or 'average' value, and a measure of variation. The

Table 1

Birthweight (kg) for 70 Premature Babies

1·11	1·18
1·20	1·31
1·34	1·05
1·66	1·32
1·80	1·27
1·62	1·50
1·27	1·40
1·57	1·38
1·48	1·21
1·40	1·19
1·19	1·56
1·36	1·30
1·22	1·41
1·16	1·02
1·20	0·95
1·55	0·99
1·20	1·04
1·05	1·35
1·21	1·65
1·36	1·60
1·20	1·60
1·40	1·58
1·20	1·43
1·05	1·44
1·26	1·90
1·35	1·97
1·55	1·35
1·39	1·40
1·62	1·75
1·42	1·69
1·57	1·40
1·87	1·89
1·34	1·07
0·93	1·15
1·42	1·50

arithmetic mean (usually abbreviated to 'mean'), median and mode usually serve as 'average' values, and the range, mean deviation, standard deviation and variance as indicators of variation.

Given raw data, the mean is the sum of the data values divided by the number of them included. From Table 1 the sum of the birthweights is 92·32 kg, and dividing by 70 we obtain the mean birthweight as 1·32 kg. This mean is the most commonly quoted average.

The median is obtained by arranging the numbers from lowest to highest and choosing the middle one, or the average of the two middle ones.

With 70 statistics arranged in rank order the median is midway between the 35th and 36th. The 35th is 1·34 kg and the 36th is 1·35 kg, so the median is $(1{\cdot}34 + 1{\cdot}35)/2 = 1{\cdot}345$ kg. The median is thus a true central value, such that there are as many below as above. In particular, one or two high extreme values which would have entered into the calculation of the mean and pushed it upwards will not affect the median, which is thus not so susceptible to extremes of variation. The calculation of the median by the method of arrangement in rank order is tedious and can be considerably simplified by being carried out after the histogram is drawn as shown in the next section.

The mode is the value which occurs most frequently. Obtaining the mode from raw data entails simply choosing the particular value which occurs most frequently. In this case there are two such weights, namely, 1·20 and 1·40 kg (a situation described as bi-modal). The worth of using the mode derives from the fact that it is the most likely observation which will occur, and it is unaffected by extremes of variation. The mode is more useful usually when it is calculated not from raw data, but after the grouping carried out to obtain the histogram described below.

The term 'average' is often applied to any one of these three measures, and since they do not necessarily coincide, the word 'average' is open to mis-use.

The Histogram

The histogram is a picture of the density of the data around the mean, median or mode. It is obtained by deciding with reference to the required detail on the limits of a number of categories or 'classes' into which the data should be sub-divided, and then counting how many observations (the 'frequency') fall into each class. The classes chosen for the data of Table 1 are shown in Table 2, together with a routine 'tally' which provides the frequencies. It is usual to have a minimum of six and a maximum of 16 classes,

Table 2

Tally for Birthweight (kg) for 70 Premature Babies

Classes[a]	Frequency
0·80→0·90	2
0·90→1·00	5
1·00→1·10	6
1·10→1·20	7
1·20→1·30	10
1·30→1·40	12
1·40→1·50	11
1·50→1·60	8
1·60→1·70	7
1·70→1·80	1
1·80→1·90	1
	Total 70

[a] → denotes up to but not including.

depending on the detail necessary. An initial analysis is best done with more detail than might finally be required. Small classes can always be merged to form broader ones.

Placing the birthweights along the horizontal (x) axis of a graph and the frequencies along the vertical (y) axis we obtain the diagram in Fig. 8, known as a histogram.

The area of each block represents the frequency with which the weights fall into the category, and since in this case the blocks have equal base lines, their heights are proportional to the frequencies. In a situation where base lines are not equal, the area (not the height) is the key to the density of the data in the category, and appropriate height adjustments need to be made. In this case the inclusion of a vertical 'frequency' scale can be misleading, and it is advantageous to write the frequencies boldly into the blocks.

Figure 8(b) differs from Fig. 8(a) in that the vertical scale shows 'relative' frequency, i.e. actual frequencies from Fig. 8(a) expressed as a proportion of the total frequencies used in Fig. 8(a). These relative frequencies can be thought of as probabilities. Thus, we would say that the probability that a randomly chosen baby from unit X has a birthweight from 1·3 to 1·4 kg is 12/70, or 0·17. In Appendix 2 we take a more detailed look at probability.

Measurements can either be 'discrete' or 'continuous'. For

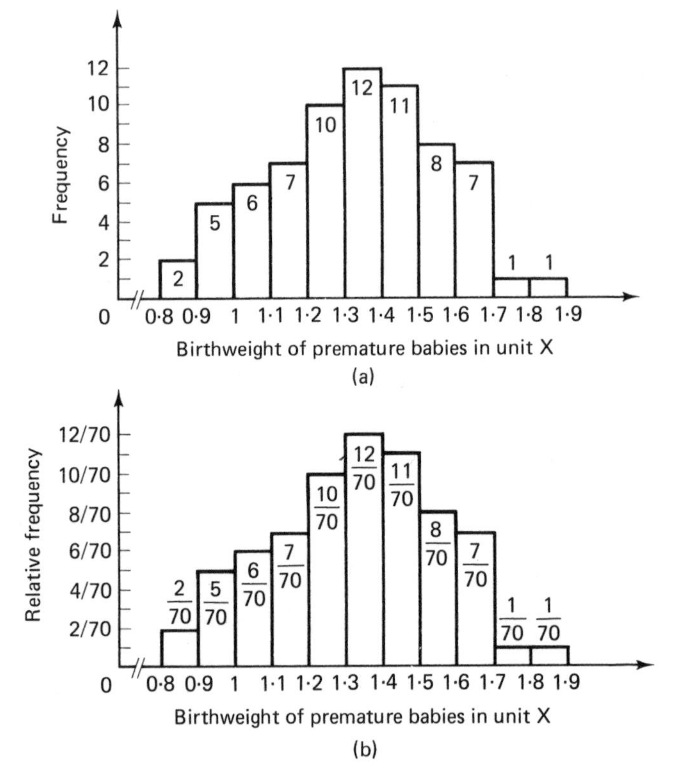

Fig. 8. Frequency histogram and relative frequency histogram for birth-weights of premature babies in unit X.

example, the number of people contracting a disease may be 18 or 19 but cannot be 18·6. Thus, the number takes 'discrete' values. In contrast, your age may be 40 or 41 or any value in between. Age is thus a 'continuous' variable as are height, weight and a multitude of other biological measures. When we draw a histogram for a continuous variable the end points of each 'block' have meaning because they are real possibilities within the data. Although we might list them in the intervals 15–24, 25–34, 35–44 and so on, we would draw them in the intervals 15–25, 25–35, 35–45, etc., being careful to allocate 25-year-olds to the 25–30 age group, the 35-year-olds to the 35–45 group and so on. We would not leave gaps between the blocks.

The number of babies born in a maternity unit is a discrete variable. The classes might be, for example: 240–249, 250–259,

260–269, etc., and there are natural gaps in the data—you cannot have 249·5 babies. The histogram blocks can either be drawn with gaps or, more commonly, the gaps can be filled thus. Taking as an example the class 260–279 this should really have a gap of one unit on each side. To fill the gap the block is drawn from 259·5 to 279·5 and the surrounding blocks are similarly handled, so that each is expanded to fill the spaces between. Figure 9(a) shows this. Of course the new end points 239·5, 259·5, 279·5, etc., no longer have real significance, and it is probably best to label the class as a grouping such as 240–259 rather than to label the actual end points, as shown in Fig. 9(b).

Approximations from Grouped Data

To complete a description of the data set it is of help to indicate the positions of the mean, median and mode. Frequently it is more efficient to obtain approximations to these *after* the histogram has been formed. Numerous formulae and computational techniques exist for these, but given the availability of pre-programmed electronic calculators, attention will not be given to formulae here. Instead, the emphasis will be placed on understanding the simplest, though computationally least sophisticated, approach to give an intuitive feeling for the nature of the calculations.

In the case of the weights it will be convenient to suppose that observations in the category 0·80 to 0·90 actually are at 0·85; all those in 0·90 to 1·00 are at 0·95, etc. These mid-points, 0·85, 0·95, etc., are called 'class marks' and the mean is obtained (approximately of course) by adding up

$$2 \times 0{\cdot}85 + 5 \times 0{\cdot}95 + 6 \times 1{\cdot}05 + 7 \times 1{\cdot}15 + 10 \times 1{\cdot}25 + 12 \times 1{\cdot}35 + 11 \times 1{\cdot}45 + 8 \times 1{\cdot}55 + 7 \times 1{\cdot}65 + 1 \times 1{\cdot}85 = 93,$$

this being a reasonable approximation to the raw data total, and dividing by 70 to obtain the *approximate* mean as $93/70 = 1{\cdot}329$, i.e. 1·33. (Compare this with the true mean obtained as 1·32 from raw data.) The median is the number which bisects the data. That is, there should be as much data above the median as below it. Having transferred the data to a histogram where areas represent visually the density of the data, the median is obtained at the point where the area is bisected, i.e. there is as much area to the left as to the right.

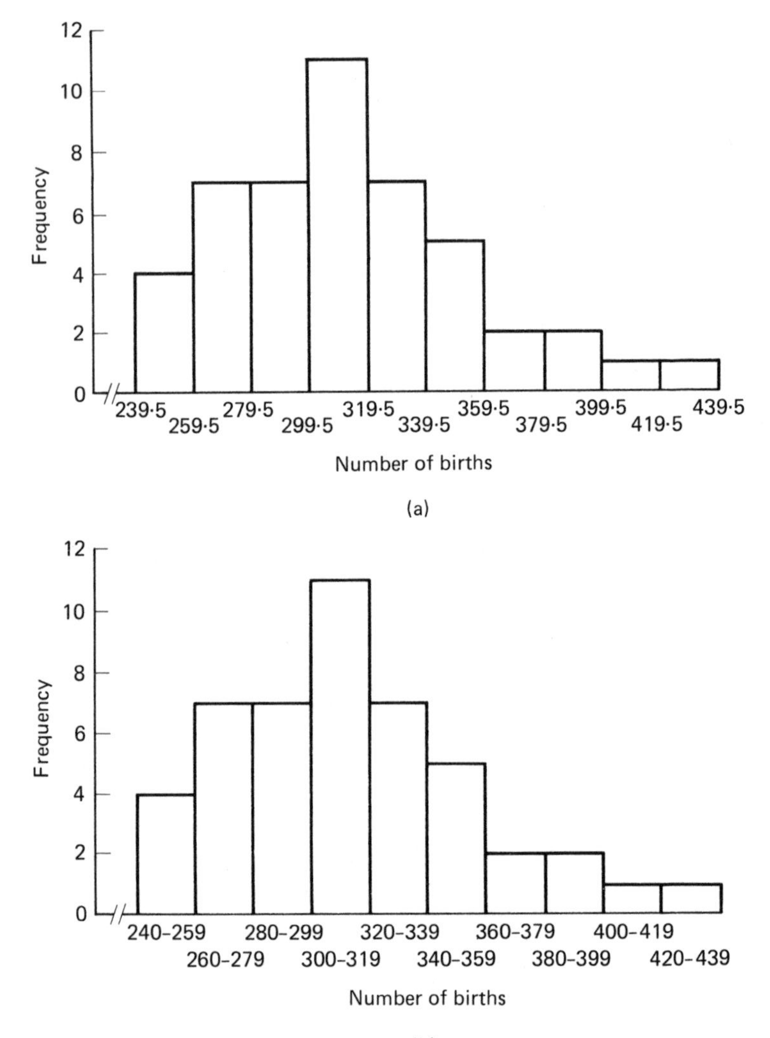

Fig. 9. (a) Number of babies born from 1 January 1976 to 31 October 1979 at a maternity hospital. (b) Number of babies born from 1 January 1976 to 31 October 1979 at a maternity hospital.

Since we have 70 weights, we regard the area under the histogram as 70, to be bisected so that 35 are on each side of the median. Starting at the extreme left hand of the histogram we add the areas of each block until we acquire around 35. Thus, at weight

1·3 kg the area to its left is 30 and at weight 1·4 kg the area to the left of it is 42. Clearly then the median lies between 1·3 and 1·4. Since we want area 35 we are short of 5 when we arrive at the point 1·3. In this class from 1·3 to 1·4 there is area 12 spread over a distance 0·1. We therefore proceed 5/12 of the way through the class, which is distance $5/12 \times 0{\cdot}1 = 0{\cdot}042$. The approximate median is then $1{\cdot}3 + 0{\cdot}042 = 1{\cdot}342$ kg.

The mode is the most frequently occurring value, or class, in this case the class 1·3 to 1·4 or class mark 1·35. (A detailed routine is available for precisely estimating the mode but the class mark is usually adequate.) The approximate measures of 'central location' are:

Mean	1·33
Median	1·34
Mode	1·35

Figure 10 shows the histogram of differences between age of onset of asthma and ages of first attendance at a paediatric asthma

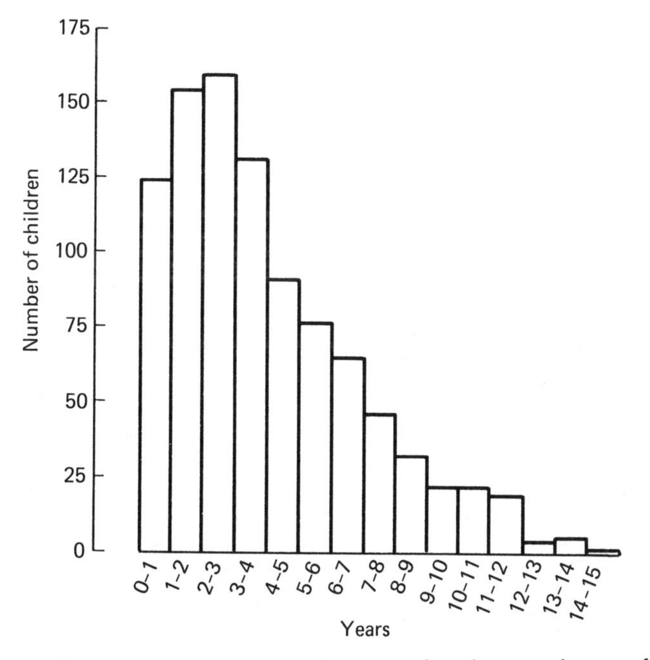

Fig. 10. Difference between age of onset of asthma and age of first attendance at the allergy clinic.

clinic. It will be noted that the histogram tails off to the right, a situation described as 'positive skew'. The mean, median and mode differ in this sort of case, being respectively 4·01, 3·31 and 2·5 years. In particular, if the mean is used as the 'average', then 60% of patients are below 'average'. Figures 11(a) and (b) show waiting times for out-patient clinic appointments, again with a positive

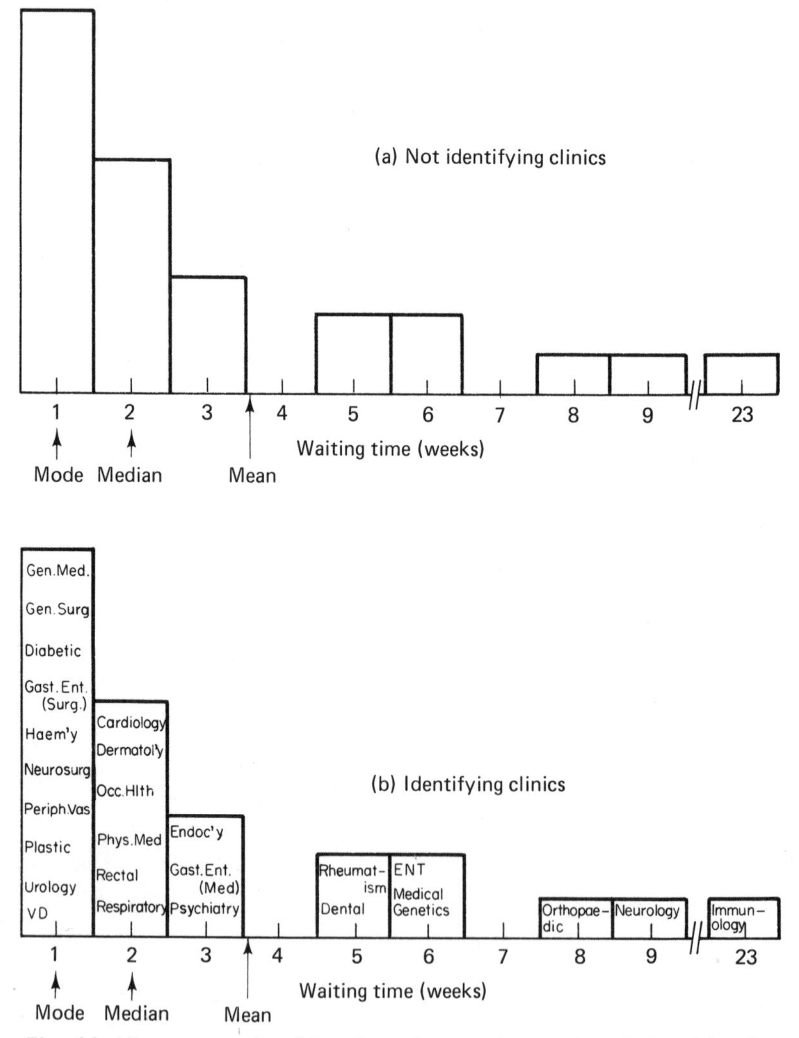

Fig. 11. Histograms of waiting times for people on a hospital waiting list.

skew and substantive differences between mean, median and mode.

It is possible to be selective in a 'political' or unfair sense when choosing which average to take. The histogram picture to supplement the chosen 'average' reduces the chance of misleading impressions.

Rates

Suppose a symptom is manifested 10% of patients in ward X, where there are 30 patients, and 20% of patients in ward Y, where there are 40 patients. The actual numbers affected are clearly three on ward X and eight on ward Y, making a total of 11 patients out of the 70 showing the symptom. This gives an overall rate of $11/70 \times 100\% = 15{\cdot}71\%$. Notice that the 'average' rate is not the mean of 10 and 20, i.e. 15%. To obtain the true percentage of 15·71 we needed first to know the actual numbers involved on each ward, then to calculate the total number affected, and finally to recalculate the percentage.

Rates of Change

If admissions to a hospital are defined as 100% in 1978 and increased by 10% to 110% in 1979, and by a further 20% to 120% of the 1979 figure in 1980, the mean percentage increase is not 15. To demonstrate this, suppose there are 1000 admissions in 1978. The rise in 1979 by 10% is to 1100, and the further increase by 20% to 1320. The total increase is 320. If we had (erroneously) averaged the 10% and 20% increases to arrive at 15%, the results of applying this average 15% increase each year would be that starting with 1000 in 1978 we would have 1150 in 1979 and 1322·5 in 1980. Thus, an extra 2·5 admissions have been 'acquired', demonstrating that the process of averaging 10% and 20% to get 15% produces an error.

The correct average to take in this case is the *geometric mean* of the two rates of increase and is calculated thus:

$$\text{Geometric mean } \% = \sqrt{110 \times 120\%}$$
$$= 114{\cdot}89\% \text{ (approx)}$$

i.e. a 14·89% increase on average

To confirm that this is correct, starting with 1000 patients in 1978 and increasing by 14·89% each year, we can predict 1148·9 in 1979 and 1320 in 1980, the correct final result.

The geometric mean of any two numbers is the square root of their product. If we have three numbers it is the cube root, with four numbers is the fourth root, and so on. The geometric mean is the correct mean to use for averaging rates of change.

Conclusions

Average can be variously defined and sometimes a particular average is more appropriate than another.

Suppose that the dosage of a drug varies according to a patient's condition. The pharmacist when asked what is the typical dose may well point to the mode, because he must make up more of this dose than any other. The hospital treasurer will be interested in the arithmetic mean dose, because when multiplied by the cost per unit he knows the total cost of this treatment. The doctor on the ward who may be uncertain of the reaction to the drug may opt to give the median dose, because, being right in the middle of the distribution, this is the safest dose in terms of minimising risk. And the Department of Health official who is monitoring the average rate of increase of use of the treatment year by year on the basis of several annual percentage increases in quantity used will need the geometric mean.

The (arithmetic) mean, median and mode are the most commonly used averages, and it is usually most helpful if a histogram showing the variation in the data is presented as back-up information. A measure of variation is a further useful statistic for monitoring and comparisons, and various possibilities are discussed in the following chapter.

4

The Standard Deviation and Other Measures of Variation

Introduction

Variation in data is often more important than the average level, especially when we realise that relatively few measurements in any distribution actually coincide with the average (however defined). We need to know when departures from average are worthy of special attention, and when they may still be considered normal.

For example, the Schwachman score for infants with cystic fibrosis may have a mean of 77, but how do we view a value of 25? Reference to the range of scores to be expected may suggest that 77 is towards an extreme, but how do we eventually judge when a deviation from the mean is typical or untypical? We need to know what the typical deviation is from the mean, and we need to take account of the density of data around the mean. Where data are concentrated near the mean, and thus have typically low deviations, then individual observations which are far out can be assessed realistically.

Using a mean without a measure of spread or dispersion strips data of a most important dimension. Using the range—the distance between the lowest and highest values—only highlights the two extreme values, and, for all the user knows, there could be nothing in between. We require a measure which combines recognition of density around the mean with ease of calculation.

Dispersion

Suppose we are informed that the mean post-operative length of hospital stay are six and seven days for matched patients of consultants A and B, respectively. Whilst having some (limited) use both clinically and for bed management, the information is incomplete because of the absence of information on patient to patient variability.

A visual comparison may be made by drawing histograms, but some quantitative indicator is required. For purposes of exposition, small numbers of patients will be considered (the sampling properties of such numbers being ignored at this point). The data are shown in Table 3. The means are six and seven days, respectively, for A and B, indicating better use of beds on average for A.

The ranges of 3 to 11 for A and 3 to 11 for B are equal, but range can be arbitrarily inflated by a single extreme, and a measure which reflects the density of the data around the mean is preferable. To this end in Table 4 we list the individual deviations from the mean, for each patient, a minus sign indicating days 'less than' average stay. Multiple occurrences, such as 4 in consultant A's data, representing high density, are retained as multiple repetitions of the deviations.

These deviations reflect dispersion and need to be summarised into a single statistic, representing an average of some sort. The mean deviation is of course zero in each case because of the mutual

Table 3

Days of Post-operative Care for each Patient of Consultants A and B

Consultant A	Consultant B
3	3
4	3
4	4
4	4
4	5
5	5
6	6
6	8
7	10
8	10
10	11
11	11
	11

Table 4

Deviations From Mean Number of Days of Post-operative Care for each Patient of Consultants A and B

Consultant A	Consultant B
−3	−4
−2	−4
−2	−3
−2	−3
−2	−2
−1	−2
0	−1
0	1
1	3
2	3
4	4
5	4
	4

cancelling of + and − signs. Two possibilities occur to overcome this problem. The first is to ignore the − signs and average the resultant 'absolute' values of the deviations. This gives

$$\text{A} \quad \frac{24}{12} = 2 \qquad \text{B} \quad \frac{38}{13} = 2{\cdot}92$$

Thus, not only does consultant B retain patients longer than consultant A, but he is also more variable in the times involved and hence B's behaviour is less predictable. In practice, of course, much larger numbers of patients would be compared, sufficient to ensure good representation; and because of the larger numbers the summary into an average deviation is all the more essential because it is more difficult to observe the variation by looking at large amounts of raw data.

The mean deviation is a useful and simple descriptive tool. An alternative possibility is to accept the − signs, and develop a way of incorporating them without ignoring them. The method is to square each deviation, as in Table 5, and then to average these squared deviations instead of the original deviations. The more dispersed is the data around the mean, the greater will be the

Table 5

Squared Deviations from Mean

	Consultant A	Consultant B
	9	16
	4	16
	4	9
	4	9
	4	4
	1	4
	0	1
	0	1
	1	9
	4	9
	16	16
	25	16
		16
Total of squared deviations	=72	=126
Mean squared deviation	$=\frac{72}{12}=6$	$=\frac{126}{13}=9{\cdot}69$

deviations, hence the greater their squares and thus the mean of their squares. Conversely, the more uniform the observations the smaller will be the deviations, their squares, and the mean of their squares. The mean squared deviation must be regarded as an index of spread which inflates with increased dispersion and deflates with uniformity of the observations. It is called variance. From a practical point of view, since the original data is in days, variance is in 'square days'. Clearly, the final step of taking the square root preserves the integrity of the original units of measurement. The figure thus obtained is the standard deviation. The results for A and B are shown in Table 6.

We may conclude that consultant B detains patients longer, and is a little less predictable (i.e. more variable) in his management of patient's length of stay than A, since A's standard deviation is less than B's.

In the case of large numbers of patients, the requirement to calculate means, variances and standard deviations assumes increasing importance as visual inspection and comparison of histograms becomes difficult.

Table 6

Summary Statistics for Consultants A and B

Statistic	Consultant A	Consultant B
Mean	6	7
Variance	6	9·69
Standard deviation	2·45	3·11
Mean deviation	2·00	2·92

The standard deviation is best understood as a close cousin of the mean deviation. It is thus convenient to think of doctor A's patients (with mean 6 days and standard deviation 2·45 days) as being detained on average 6 days, but the average difference from 6 days for any patient is 2·45 days. We are thus treating the standard deviation as though it is a mean deviation, its 'cousin'. The standard deviation is, in general, to be preferred to the mean deviation because it has fuller mathematical development and possibilities, has many convenient documented properties, and is available on inexpensive calculators at the touch of a key. Its importance in sampling is fundamental.

We conclude by saying that a minimum acceptable set of descriptive statistics for any batch of data is the mean and standard deviation, and a histogram provides an excellent visual summary and indicator of density about the mean. In certain circumstances the mode and median are useful, but they are limited from the point of view of possible mathematical development. The median is important when data have meaning only in terms of rank order. This type of data might be assigned as the result of (subjectively) rating the condition of a group of patients, from worst to best. Though a scale may be used, the numbers would only have ordinal significance, and the median, i.e. the middle value, would have more use than the mean because position is more meaningful than numerical value. The area of statistics known as non-parametric statistics deals with data which has only rank order value, and is discussed in Chapter 7.

Use of the Standard Deviation

The standard deviation is useful because two large batches of data can be instantly compared for 'variability'; or one batch can be analysed at different points in time. There are a number of inferences that can be made about data when the data and histogram are not available but the mean and standard deviation are known. Tchebbycheff's theorem is of interest here. For example, one of the results of this theorem is that at least 75% of the observations in any distribution lie within a distance two times the standard deviation on either side of the mean, and at least 88·9% lie within three standard deviations of the mean. The importance of the 'at least' should not be overlooked. (The theorem states that for k exceeding 1, at least $1-(1/k^2)$ of the observations in any histogram, whatever its shape, lie within k times the standard deviation from the mean. Our examples above related to $k=2$ and $k=3$, respectively.) Frequently, *all* the observations lie within three times the standard deviation. We have mentioned that Tchebbycheff applies where the shape of the histogram is unknown. When some information is available, we can be more precise. Frequently it is known by experience that the histogram is bell shaped around the mean. This is the 'normal' or Gaussian distribution. Here, instead of the Tchebbycheff result which gave *at least 75%* of data within two standard deviations of the mean we can say that, the closer to the perfect theoretical 'bell shape', the more confident can we be that exactly 95% of the data lie in this interval. And for the interval three standard deviations on either side of the mean, we can say that, not only at least 88·9% as in Tchebbycheff, but 99·7% of the data are here. Thus, broadly speaking, knowledge of the standard deviation helps 'place' the distribution and its density. A final useful fact is that just over 2/3 (68%) of the data in a normal distribution lies within a distance equal to the standard deviation on either side of the mean. These percentages are illustrated in Fig. 12.

It will be noticed that we speak of two standard deviations. The standard deviation is the unit of measurement in the histogram, and enables us to compare the relative positions of points in histograms which are on different scales or in different units. Thus, consider two normal distributions A and B with measurements as shown in Figs. 13 and 14, respectively, and as follows:

A—Mean, 5	B—Mean, 50
Standard deviation, 2·5	Standard deviation, 2·5

It will first be noticed that the standard deviations, though equal, show that A is relatively more dispersed than B, since its standard

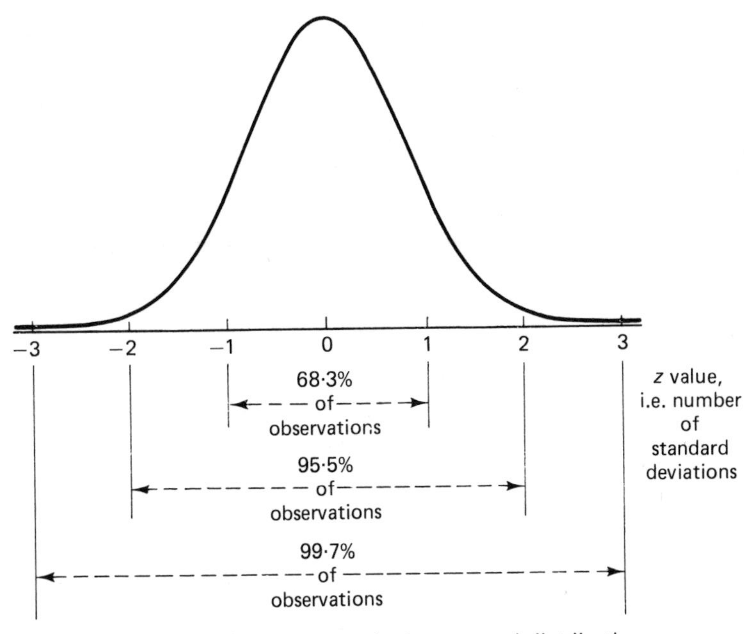

Fig. 12. Observation density in a normal distribution.

deviation of 2·5 is 50% of its mean value, compared with 5% for B. This measure,

$$\left(\frac{\text{Standard deviation}}{\text{Mean}}\right) \times 100$$

is the coefficient of variation, a useful measure of relative dispersion for situations where we wish to make comparisons of

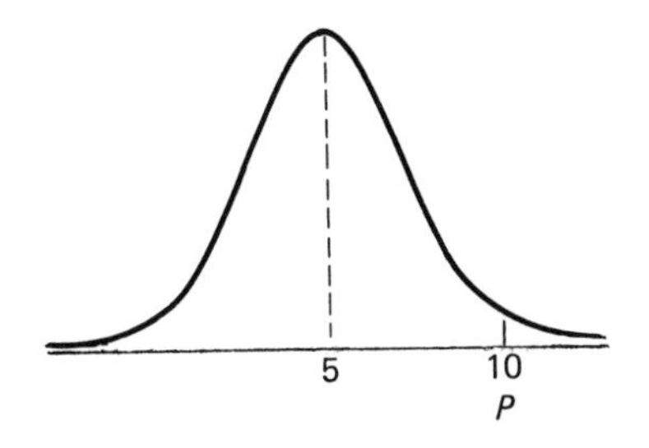

Fig. 13. A normal distribution with mean=5 and standard deviation =2·5.

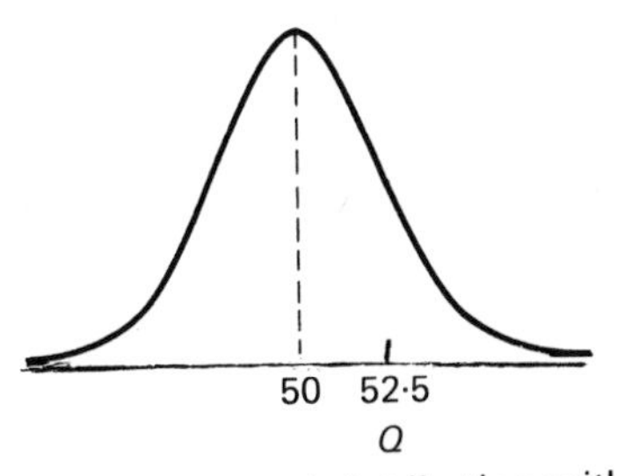

Fig. 14. A normal distribution with mean=50 and standard deviation =2·5.

spread when the means are dissimilar. Now consider points P and Q on each of the normal distributions A and B in Figs. 13 and 14 and the question of which is relatively higher in relation to the mean.

Point P is a distance 5 from the mean, which is twice the standard deviation. Q is a distance 2·5, which is one times the standard deviation. P is thus a relatively higher point than Q. Now consider a normal distribution mean 0, standard deviation 1. This is the *standard* normal distribution of Fig. 15. P′ at scale point 2 is the equivalent of P, and Q′ at scale point 1 is equivalent to Q. By equivalent we mean 'are relatively the same point in the distribution'. And by this we mean that, for example, in the case of Q, approximately 16% of values exceed it, and for P, approximately 2·5%. It is a feature of the normal distribution that as long as 'equivalent' points are being considered, the percentage of data to the left and right of each point is the same whatever the scale of the histogram. The standard normal distribution has all such percentages tabulated. Thus, in the case of a non-standard normal distribution, all that is required is to find its equivalent points, such as P′, Q′, and then the tables make available the percentage of observations above or below this value. Thus, for P′, 2·5% lie above it. Hence this is true for P. Another way of saying this is that there

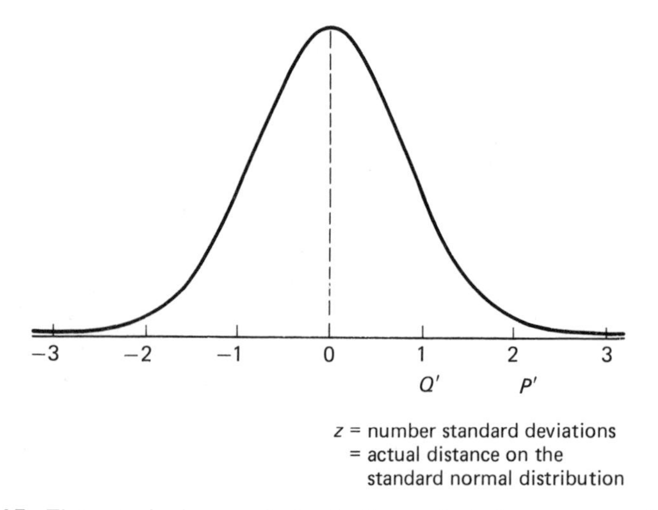

Fig. 15. The standard normal distribution, which has a mean=0 and standard deviation=1.

is a probability of 2·5% or 0·025 that any value selected at random from the distribution is above P.

The standard properties of the normal distribution are fundamental in making inferences on the basis of samples.

Formal *z* 'Score'

Following on from the previous comments on the standard deviation as the unit of measurement, this operates formally in the following way. Given a scale on which we have a point x, mean m and standard deviation σ, we say that the 'equivalent' point on the standard normal distribution is

$$\frac{x-m}{\sigma}$$

and this is referred to as z. In words, it is the number of standard deviations which x lies away from m. The statistic z is fundamental when we discuss sampling properties of the mean. Appendix 3a shows a table of the areas (i.e. probabilities) under the standard normal distribution, and hence under any normal distribution for any value of z.

Conclusions

Variation in data is usually more important than the average level. Several measures of variation are available, of which the standard deviation is the most useful. It is particularly important when we evaluate the worth of sampling results, and begin to test hypotheses. The descriptive uses of the standard deviation and its ease of calculation using modern technology renders it an essential complement to measures of average in common use.

In closing we may now answer a question put earlier in this chapter. 'In infants with cystic fibrosis where the mean Schwachman score is 77 how do we view a score of 25?' The answer depends on the standard deviation, which when measured is found to be 22. The difference between 77 and 25 can now be meaningfully expressed in terms of the number of standard deviations it represents. The calculation gives

$$z = (25\text{–}77) \div 22 = -2{\cdot}36$$

By any standards therefore the score of 25 is somewhat extreme, and if it is known that these scores are approximately normally distributed, a z value of 2·36 puts 25 into the lowest 0·9% of the distribution. Such a score happens only 9 times in 1000.

5

Sampling Principles and Confidence Intervals

Introduction

Samples are an important part of life. We commonly make decisions about matters ranging from the mundane purchase of apples to the major expenditure on a car on the basis of a sample of information which reaches us. It is usually impossible or impractical to study all members of any population, whether they are patients, bacteria, tablets, syringes or even doctors themselves. Sometimes the very act of examination is in itself destructive of a desirable property of the object being examined, and to study all members of the group would render the whole 'population' useless. Sterile supplies constitute such a case. The act of examination renders them useless.

Samples are used in place of censuses (i.e. complete enumerations) because they are cheaper, quicker to obtain and analyse, frequently more accurate than a census because the smallness of the sample permits good 'control' over the process of sampling, and sometimes inevitable because populations are so large or inaccessible that there is no way of studying every member in a reasonable period of time.

The basic elements which make up populations are called sampling units. Thus, a human population is made up of individual people, each of whom is a 'unit'. Sample studies attempt to collect together a group of units to make the sample. Sometimes these units are reached by mail, telephone, personal interview at the home, consultation in surgery or hospitals, and so on.

Planning a sampling study is the most important step. Poor planning can render an expensive study useless. The first step in planning is to define the population of interest, and if possible obtain a list of its members—a 'sampling frame'. The type of sample must be decided, together with the method of obtaining responses, such as the use of a questionnaire filled in by, say the patient or the interviewer, or physical measurements and who should do them. The best types of samples are sometimes referred to as 'random samples' or scientific samples. There are other samples such as 'convenience samples' which include anyone who happens to be convenient to the study, and judgement samples which include those members judged to be desirable for inclusion. Statistical theory applies only to random samples. Consequently, no legitimate conclusions on, for example, error bounds can be inferred for non-random samples.

A choice of analytical method, of statistical tests to be conducted and of relationships sought should be made before a sample study is begun. Choosing any of these once the results start to come available can produce innocent or intentional bias towards a desired conclusion.

The choice of sample size is important. The common myth that a sample twice as large as another is twice as good is not true. To be 'twice as good'—which we may take to mean to halving the sampling error of our results—actually requires a quadrupling of sample size. To be 'three times as good' requires a sample size to be increased to nine times its original size. These results, of course, apply to simple random sampling and are not intuitively obvious. We return to them later in this chapter. It is possible to improve precision of a simple random sample by switching to a stratified random sample of the same size. Stratification is discussed shortly. Having come this far—making decisions on all planning matters—the next stage is data collection. It is essential that strict control over the procedure for data collection is enforced, and that when a 'control' group forms one sample and a 'trial' group forms another for comparison (see Chapter 7), the patients are allocated randomly, without judgemental factors interfering—to the appropriate group. Where a questionnaire is administered to patients, then the questions need pre-testing and very careful ordering and design. A manual of questionnaire design is invaluable (e.g. Oppenheim A. W. (1966). *Questionnaire Design & Attitude Measurement.* London: Heinemann). Non-response or 'dropping out' by certain sections of the population or sample can present real problems of bias and important decisions need to be made in the manner of dealing with such omissions. Data handling and preparation procedures need to be carefully controlled for the final stage of a sampling study, where we analyse the data and draw some conclusions.

If a computer program is to be used to analyse the questionnaires, then they need efficient design so that coding the responses is simple, efficient and easily read by the person who 'punches up' the data for the computer. Procedures need to be designed for checking the 'keypunching'.

Finally, when all planning and data collection and 'arithmetic' is over, the 'report' needs to be drawn up. The statistical conclusions should be phrased in a manner that permits others to readily evaluate the work. Sample design, sample size, questions levels of significance and of confidence, etc., etc., need careful listing for this vital final stage.

Survey Errors

The two main types of error in a sample study are 'statistical error' (or 'sampling error') and non-statistical error (or 'non-sampling error'). The former is almost inevitable when studying a small group extracted from a population. It would be incredibly unlikely that the members in the small group (i.e. sample) would be a perfect microcosm of the population. There is almost certain to be a difference between the sample value measured and the true population counterpart, however good our procedures and sampling method. This inevitable difference is statistical or sampling error. Non-statistical or non-sampling error is primarily procedural—it relates to the manner in which the observation is made and thus in theory can be minimised by controls over the interviewers, methods of data collection, and so on. The easiest understood example of non-statistical error is an error in a physiological measurement such as blood pressure, due to sphygmomanometer fault, or operator fault. Another example would be when a patient being interviewed for the study deliberately concealed some relevant factor, such as exact age. This latter can frequently be overcome by getting date of birth, which, if there is hesitation, indicates some quick arithmetic faking is being attempted.

Sometimes the purpose of the study needs to be 'concealed' to obtain information which minimises non-statistical error. For example, to choose a patient at random from a register and to ask a number of direct questions about venereal disease will almost certainly result in substantial non-response and hence error in conclusions. The study may have to be 'couched' in terms of general health, and subtly pick up all the relevant facts on venereal disease at different points on the questionnaire to make them appear unrelated. In this sort of study, further non-statistical error can come from the attitude of the interviewer which may induce bias. Rephrasing of questions may take place to minimise embarrassment, and unwittingly bias the results. Similarly, vocal emphasis of words or phrases can happen, with biasing effects on the results. In the following sections the only errors we discuss are statistical errors. In 'real' surveys it is the non-statistical errors which are crucial. No sampling survey should be conducted without reference to a statistician and a standard reference on surveys. Surveys are an area for trained and highly skilled professionals. Though they may *appear* easy to do—'anyone can ask questions'—is a frequent comment, we need only mention that to a layman, administering a general anaesthetic also appears easy, especially when he sees it carried out in hospital 'soap operas' on television.

Types of Sample

We now will briefly discuss six types of sample, and focus carefully on the last four. The main sample designs in common use are convenience samples, judgement samples, simple random samples, systematic random samples, stratified random samples, and cluster samples.

A convenience sample is just that: convenient. A doctor in general practice may wish to study the effect of a drug on his patients. All patients who present with a relevant sympton during the next eight weeks may be 'convenient' to be the sample. They may be uncontrolled and totally unrepresentative of all patients to whom the results are to be extended. But they are convenient to deal with and are a 'convenience sample'. If the results are to be generalised no further than the subpopulation of patients who present to this doctor in this location with the predefined set of symptoms, then the convenience sample may be of local use.

A judgement sample is obtained using the discretion or judgement of the interviewer. In commercial market research, for example, an interviewer may be given a 'quota' of respondents to find. For example, the sample may need 50 'middle class' females of child bearing age. The actual selection is up to the interviewer, and potentially there is bias in this method. The more approachable or attractive members of society would be expected to predominate. When a very small sample is essential, or when special skills are important to decide whether sampling units display a representative mix of qualities, then the judgement sample might find medical use. The quality of such a sample reflects greatly on the person who selects it.

The simple random sample allows each elementary unit an equal chance (or probability) of being chosen. The term probability sample is also used for this type of sample. It is desirable that each element in the sampling frame be given a number. Either a computer based random number generator should be used to give a list of numbers to be the sample, or a random number table can supply the list cheaply and quickly. Suppose a general practitioner's list is numbered 1 to 3000 and a simple random sample of 100 patients is to be chosen. If a random number table gives, say five digit numbers, we would be interested only in the first four digits which could give us numbers 0000 to 9999. Any in the range 0001 to 3000 are relevant and we would take as our sample the first 100 of these, ignoring the 0000 and any from 3001 to 9999 inclusive. If the same number occurred more than once, its repetitions would be excluded and extra 'make-up' numbers substituted. It does not matter how a random number table is read—left to right, bottom to top—as long as this is specified beforehand and not altered to specifically include any members of the sampling frame.

Sometimes it is not possible or convenient to number every member of a population. This would be so when a full sampling frame cannot be obtained. When people are to be interviewed at home or in the street, the simple random sample using a random number table may dictate waiting for the 99th person to pass by, or walking to the 99th house on a block, when several perfectly eligible respondents could be found in between. It may thus be convenient to simplify the collection of our data if we use, for example, every tenth passerby, or every tenth house, or every tenth name on a list. Interviewers find this an easy system to operate. The first respondent may be chosen using a random number. Thereafter, all inclusions in the sample are automatic.

Depending on the size of the sample, size of the population and organisational and economic factors, the interval, whether we take the 10th, 15th, 20th, etc., name on the list after the first, is decided.

If there is periodicity in the list this can cause bias. For example, a list of houses by occupant may read:

No.1—Mr Jones
Mrs Jones
No.2—Mr Smith
Mrs Smith
.
.
.
No.37—Mr Black
Mrs Black
.
.
.

Suppose we take every tenth name, starting randomly. The alternate scores listed may result in an all-male sample or an all-female sample, depending on where we start. This is a somewhat extreme example, but nevertheless, periodicities do sometimes occur and can give an unrepresentative sample. Provided we are satisfied that our systematic random sample is unbiased, we treat it statistically as though it is a random sample.

Frequently we will know in advance of a study that the response we will obtain will differ according to some characteristic of the population such as sex or age. Accordingly, we may not wish to leave to chance the inclusion of representatives of each sex or age group in our sample. After all, a simple random sample of people in general could accidentally turn out to be all male and over 65 years old, when we really want a mixed sex group ranging from say 15 to 85. By deliberately deciding on strata in advance, we reduce the potential variability of our samples, and can increase the precision of the results. We are, in effect, making sure that extreme samples will not show up. Provided the criterion for making the stratification is relevant to the object of the survey, the extra work will be worthwhile. If, for example, we are studying a podiatric problem and stratify by whether people are blond or dark haired, we will probably have stratified in vain, because there is no known association between foot problems and hair colour. On the other hand, if we stratify first by sex, and then within each sex by broad age groups, we may make useful improvements to our sampling precision, as well as providing statistics by sex and age group as a bonus. To obtain an overall sample statistic, such as the proportion with a specified characteristic from a stratified sample, requires combining the estimates from each stratum into an overall estimate. The strata statistics are appropriately weighted according to their importance. It is desirable that strata be as homogeneous internally as possible, but as different from each other as possible. This sort of design yields good sample results.

The cluster sample is obtained by first subdividing the population into groupings, such as neighbourhoods or districts, and then choosing at random a group of clusters to be the sample. For example, in the UK for a study of hospitals, a cluster might be a health district. From the list of all existing districts we may choose 50, and within each of the 50 would carry out a census type study, looking at every hospital in each of the 50 clusters. The justification for this is economic and logistical. We might acquire, say, 300 hospitals for our study if there are six per cluster. An alternative way of obtaining 300, for example by random sampling, would produce 300 scattered throughout the country, causing considerble data collection expense, making control difficult, and taking much more time to conduct the study. However, clusters can be idiosyncratic. In certain clusters there may be a tendency for certain ethnic or socioeconomic groupings to predominate. Particular medical conditions may have a greater prevalence. There is no guarantee that all the clusters taken together will be adequately representative of the population. Whereas in stratified random sampling the strata are chosen deliberately to represent the population and all groups are represented, in cluster sampling the clusters are chosen for economic convenience. Bias is a very real possibility in cluster sampling.

More complex sampling schemes than those described can be carried out. In particular, 'multi stage' methods are used by statisticians. Essentially they all develop from the methods described in this chapter. For example, in a cluster sampling situation we may first divide the population into clusters and randomly sample 50 clusters. This completes stage 1. We may then stratify each cluster and conduct stratified sampling within the cluster. This is stage 2, and differs from our earlier description of cluster sampling because we are not taking a census within each cluster. Complex multi-stage designs need expert statistical assistance *before* implementation.

In the following analysis when we talk of samples we mean simple random samples, where each member of the population has an equal chance of being included in the sample. The method by which the random sample members are chosen precludes human judgement and is carried out by some electronic or mechanical method which is independent of the operator. We exclude samples of convenience or where the judgement of the interviewer is crucial, with the possibility of bias, and where undoubtedly the more 'approachable' or vociferous members of the public would be included. For these types of sample, the results of this chapter are not applicable. For the sake of clarity and simplicity we also do not include results for stratified or cluster sampling.

The Normal Distribution

Suppose that from a very large and carefully defined population a random sample of people is chosen and given a lung function test, producing the following FEV scores as a percentage of expected: 63, 88, 86, 21 and 93, with sample mean calculated as 70·2. Another random sample is then chosen, and the values which result are: 89, 72, 43, 36, and 98, with sample mean 67·6. This is clearly different from our first value. Repetition 100 times of this process yields a list of such means, which are grouped into classes giving the histogram of Fig. 16. It is noticeably the familiar 'bell shape' known as the normal (or Gaussian) distribution. This histogram is known as 'the sampling distribution of the mean', and in general as we increase the number of means included, and as we increase the sample size, the more perfect will be the resulting normal distribution curve. This result, which applies to several types of sample statistics, in particular the sample mean and a sample proportion with a specified attribute, is known as the 'Central Limit Theorem' and is basic to the understanding of sampling and hypothesis testing.

The diagrammatic presentation in Fig. 17 should make the process clear. The symbols in use in the diagram are those most commonly used.

The build up of the sample means into a normal distribution

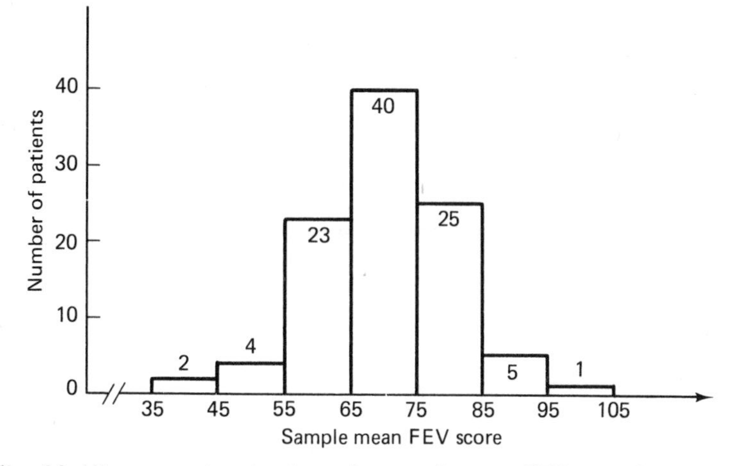

Fig. 16. Histogram showing how the sample mean FEV score from a lung function test is distributed.

does *not* depend on the original population being normally distributed—its histogram could be any shape. However, to make inferences about how much in 'error' our sample mean is in relation to the true mean, we need to know something about the spread of possible sample means. Spread is measured by standard deviation, and when we are working on the list of all possible sample means, their particular standard deviation is referred to as the 'standard error' of the mean, often abbreviated as SEM. There are two main factors which affect the standard error of the mean. The first of these is the variability in the original population, and the second is the sample size.

If the original population is very dispersed, i.e. quite heterogeneous, then clearly this will be reflected in random samples drawn from it, so that a random sample could contain all 'high' values and give a 'high' mean, or equally could contain all 'low' values and generate a 'low' mean. Another way of saying the original population is 'very dispersed about its mean' is to say it has a high standard deviation, and in this case the standard error of the mean will be large. Conversely, if the original population is fairly uniform (i.e. has a small standard deviation), there will be little variation from sample mean to sample mean, and hence the standard error of the mean will be small. There is in fact a simple proportionality, such that the standard error of the sample means

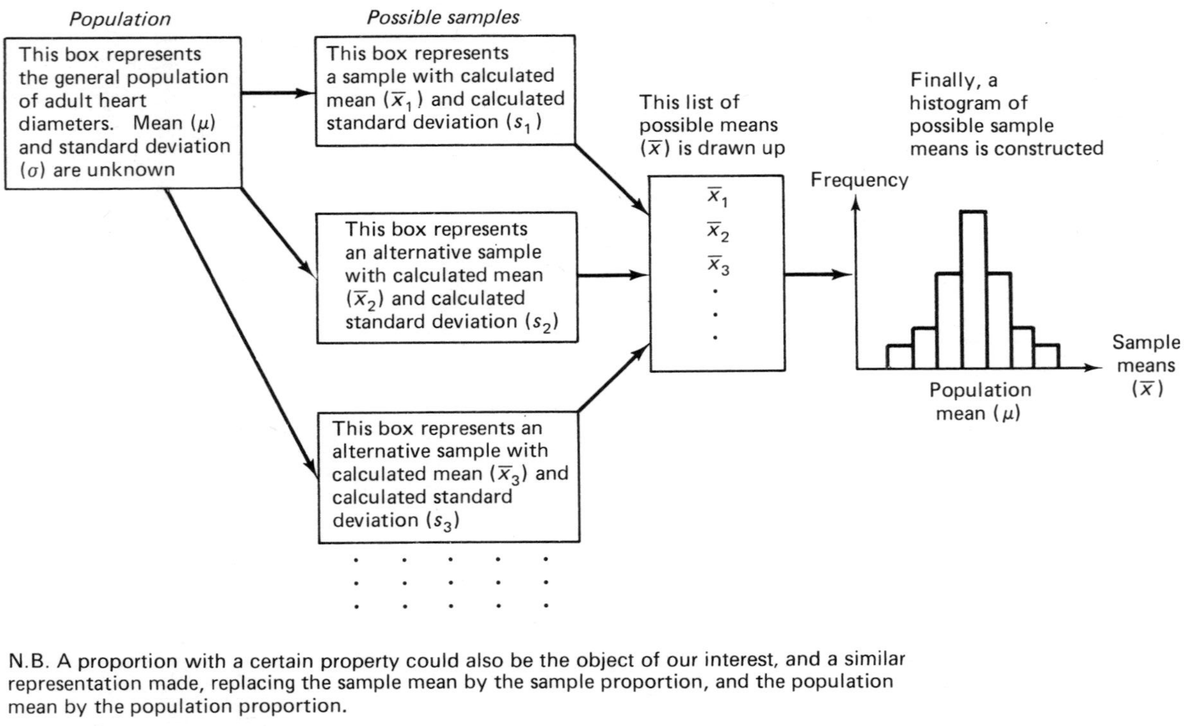

N.B. A proportion with a certain property could also be the object of our interest, and a similar representation made, replacing the sample mean by the sample proportion, and the population mean by the population proportion.

Fig. 17. A diagrammatic representation of the situation resulting in the histogram of sample means.

is directly proportional to the standard deviation of the population.

If the number in the sample is large, one would expect its mean to have a good chance of being close to the true mean, i.e. one would expect the distribution of sample means to be dense around the true mean. Conversely, if the sample is small, one would expect the samples to be more variable and less dense around the true mean. Thus, one would *intuitively* expect that, for example, doubling sample size would halve the standard error of the sample mean; tripling sample size should reduce standard error to 1/3, i.e. an inverse relation. The correct result is that standard error of the sample mean is inversely proportional to the *square root of the sample size.* What actually happens, in brief, is that to halve the standard error we need to take a sample four times as large. To reduce standard error to 1/3 we need to take a sample nine times as large, and to reduce, say to 1/4, the sample needs to be magnified 16 times in size. The actual formula reads:

$$\text{Standard error of sample mean} = \frac{\text{Standard deviation of population}}{\text{Square root of sample size}}$$

This result has implications for sampling as shown in the following example. Consider a sample of 64 patients from a population with standard deviation 10. The reliability of the sample mean depends on the histogram of possible means that could have arisen in sampling with sample size 64. We assess this reliability by hoping for a low standard error of the mean, which will be proportional to 1/8.

Suppose now further precision is required and thus the sample is increased four-fold to 256 patients, involving over four times as much medical or surgical time, more laboratory and nursing work, etc. The effect on the precision of the results is to make the standard error of the mean reduce to being proportional to 1/16, i.e. a reduction by a factor of only two for an increase of sample size by a factor of four, underlining the fact that to halve the statistical error in random sampling you need to quadruple the sample.

The Central Limit Theorem can be expressed in several ways, but for our purposes we may summarise with the statement that the means of random samples from large populations will be normally distributed around the original population mean with standard deviation inversely proportional to the square root of sample size and directly proportional to the population standard deviation. As sample size increases the normal curve becomes more perfect, but the result is often usable even for small sample sizes above about five. We may now use the properties of the normal curve referred to earlier in Chapter 4.

The Concept of a Confidence Interval

We can say, for example, that since 99·7% of values under any normal curve lie within three times the standard deviation from the mean, in our case 99·7% of possible sample means lie within a distance three times the standard error of the mean from the correct value. Putting this another way, we can be virtually certain (99·7%) that *any* random sample mean has an error no greater than three times the standard error. If we calculate the interval, which starts at the mean minus three times standard error and goes up to the mean plus three times the standard error, we can be 99·7% confident that within it lies the true mean. This interval is referred to as a 99·7% confidence interval.

Alternatively, we can say that 95% of values of a normal curve lie within approximately two times the standard deviation from the mean. Thus, 95% of the possible sample means differ by no more than twice the standard error from the true mean. For any random sample mean there is a 95% chance that it displays a maximum error of twice the standard error. The interval, starting from the sample mean minus twice the standard error and finishing at the sample mean plus twice the standard error, should contain the true population mean with the probability 0·95. This interval is referred to as a 95% confidence interval.

Any percentage confidence interval can be computed in this way by deciding on the percentage, say 75, using the tables of the normal curve to discover that 75% lie within $z = 1{\cdot}15$ standard deviations of the mean, and then setting the 75% confidence interval as the sample mean plus or minus 1·15 times the standard error. All that needs to be found is the appropriate z, in this case 1·15. Finally, it should be noted that confidence intervals for the proportion, the difference between means and the difference between two proportions, are amenable to a similar treatment.

The standard error of the mean is calculated by dividing the population standard deviation by the square root of sample size. However, the standard deviation of the original population is not likely to be known. If a similar study is available an estimate of the population standard deviation from this might be used. Alternatively, since the sample 'reflects' the population, the sample standard deviation may be used as an estimate. In 'large' samples, above 30, this presents no problems, but for samples under 30 the reliability of the sample standard deviation comes into question and an alternative procedure is required.

Because of the unreliability of the sample standard deviation in samples containing less than 30 members, we cannot be as sure that the confidence interval, as worked out above, will actually contain the true mean with the stated probability. To retain the level of probability for our statement we need to widen the interval. This is done in the 95% case by multiplying the standard error by a number slightly larger than the z value of 2. The 'replacement' is known as a 't' value, and there is a different value according to each sample size under 30. In the 99·7% case we would replace the $3 \times$ standard error by the appropriate value from t tables. We do, however, need to make the assumption that the original population is normally distributed before we can go to the use of t tables for our confidence intervals. We need to use 't' only when samples are small *and* the population standard deviation is estimated from the sample. If we had an alternative reliable estimate then we would not make the transition from z confidence interval to the t confidence interval.

Conclusions

Random samples are sometimes preferable to complete enumeration (i.e. census), and sometimes inevitable, as for example with potentially infinite population sizes. Very large samples may actually not be rewarded with 'better' results than small samples. First, it is more difficult to control the quality of the data being collected, and second doubling the sample size does not halve the standard error in simple random sampling. To achieve a halving of standard error requires a quadrupling of the sample, and the extra time and costs may be unjustified in terms of the improved results. Reduction in standard error for a given sample size can usually be achieved by stratifying the sample, provided that this is done by a factor relevant to the object of our study.

When sample results are quoted it is advisable to qualify them with information on method of sampling (e.g. simple random), the size of the sample, and error bounds either in the form of a standard error, or a confidence interval.

To be able to assess sampling error, the method of sampling needs to be random. Non-random methods whilst being economical do not permit valid estimates of error.

Non-sampling error (such as interviewer bias) is potentially very damaging to sample results, but good procedures and controls can minimise non-sampling error.

No survey should be conducted without prior reference to a manual on survey design, and a discussion of the study—in particular the method of analysis of results—with a statistician or computer analyst. Five minutes of consultation can prevent invalid methodology from proceeding, and can save weeks of unnecessary work.

6

Statistical Tests and the Concept of Significance

Introduction

The concept of the confidence interval applies to sampling statistics in general but is used primarily for means, proportions, the difference between the means of two groups, and the difference between the proportions with a particular characteristic in two groups. The confidence interval is our guide to the error due to sampling, providing a range within which we should expect to find the true population parameter with a specified high level of confidence.

We use confidence intervals when we do not have a preconceived idea as to the value of the underlying population parameter. In situations where we do have specific ideas about parameters, our objective changes to testing hypotheses about parameter values. The first part of this chapter is concerned with 'parametric' tests, and later we move on to situations where we are testing hypotheses which are not about particular parameters—a branch of statistics known as non-parametric testing.

A Simple Hypothesis Test

As an example of a simple parametric test suppose a new feed additive is given to a random sample of 32 low birth-weight babies. There is in existence a 'standard' feeding regime which is known to produce over the first eight weeks of life a mean gain in weight of 170 g per week. For the new additive the mean weight gain is expected to exceed the existing 170 g. We take a somewhat cautious and conservative approach to testing the additive by setting up a hypothesis which nullifies the claim to improvement. This hypothesis—the 'null hypothesis'—states that the mean weight gain is still 170 g. Only if the sample data seem inconsistent with 170 g will the null hypothesis be rejected in favour of the alternative hypothesis, which in this case would be that there is an increase in weight. The underlying approach in hypothesis testing is always that a new method will not be accepted as improving on the old unless the sample demonstrates this in a convincing manner.

Assuming that the 'old' mean weight gain still applies, then sample means would be distributed around 170 g with a standard error calculated as the standard deviation of the population divided by the square root of sample size. The sample has 32 members, and with sample mean 203 the standard deviation of the population is known from previous experience as 65. (In the sample the standard deviation is 67·4, which would be used to estimate the population standard deviation if the latter were not known.) Hence, the standard error of the mean is $65 \div \sqrt{32} = 11{\cdot}49$. The distribution of sample means expected under the null hypothesis is shown in Fig. 18, and we would now ask whether the sample mean value fits into this distribution in a way which encourages us to think that the sample mean is a typical member of this distribution. If it is a typical member, then the new feeding method has not produced a sample value that differs significantly from those we expect under the old method. On the other hand, if the sample

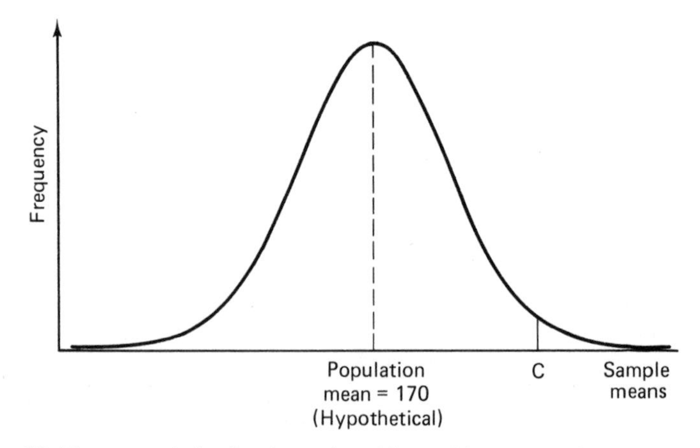

Fig. 18. The normal distribution—the ultimate histogram of sample means.

mean is substantially larger than the values in Fig. 18, or is very clearly in the upper (right) tail, we may begin to think that a real increase in weight gain is being accomplished. We need to decide on a cut-off point, such as C in Fig. 18, such that if our sample mean falls to the right (above) C, then we reject the null hypothesis of 'no change' and accept the alternative of some improvement. The position of C depends on the 'significance level' of the test, which in turn is a matter for judgement and experience, although conventionally the significance level is chosen at 5% (i.e. 0·05), or less often at either 10% (i.e. 0·01) or 1% (i.e. 0·001). Suppose we decide that the level is to be 5%. The point C is located such that 5% of all sample means that could be generated if the null hypothesis were true would exceed C. This means that an area, or probability, 0·05 lies to the right of C, and using tables of the standard normal distribution, we can read off the z value at C as 1·645. That is, C lies a distance 1·645 times the standard error to the right of the hypothesised mean. We now look at our sample mean and calculate its z value as $(203-170)\div 11{\cdot}9=2{\cdot}77$. The sample mean thus has a greater z value than that at C, and falls to the right of C. We would conclude that it appears not to be consistent with the null hypothesis that the mean is 170, and we reject the null hypothesis. The alternative hypothesis of an improvement has thus found support in the sample, at the 5% significance level.

There is, however, the possibility that the original 170 mean is still operative, but quite by chance one of its more extreme samples, falling in the upper tail, has occurred. The probability of this is 0·05, and we chose to designate this section of the distribution as being inconsistent with 170. The null hypothesis of 170 is then incorrectly rejected, and we have committed a type I error. Since the probability is 0·05 or less that the null hypothesis will legitimately give a sample in its own rejection region, the test is usually qualified with a probability statement to the effect, namely $P \leqslant 0{\cdot}05$.

It may intuitively be felt that a reduction in the significance level to 0·01 would be preferred. However, the 'cost' of this reduction will be an increase in the probability of an 'opposite' error, namely accepting the null hypothesis when it is false—a type II error. For example, if the true mean unknown to the investigator is now 175, then a real improvement over 170 has been obtained. But the chance that 175 will generate a value which is consistent with 170 and falls in the acceptance region for 170 is high. In this case 170 would be erroneously accepted, and a type II error thus is committed. A potentially useful treatment may then be discarded. For any postulated true mean, such as 175, and for a particular sample size, we can measure the probability of a type II error, and hence reveal how discriminating our testing procedure really is. A graph of the probability of accepting the value specified by the null hypothesis against the possible true mean is known as the 'operating characteristic curve'.

The test we have just described was a 'one-tail' test—so called because we had an alternative hypothesis relating to an improvement, a move into the upper tail—of the mean. Sometimes we may not have a clear idea of what we are expecting. A trial may be expected to produce change, but we cannot say in advance of taking the sample whether results would be expected to be in the upper or lower tail of the sampling distribution in order to reject the null hypothesis. Accordingly, we are prepared to look in both tails, and the level of significance, say 5%, is split equally between the tails.

Just as we may make a hypothesis test on a mean, so other parameters such as the proportion with a particular characteristic, or the difference between the means of two samples, or the difference between the proportions in two samples can be tested using the same type of theory. An example relating to a proportion is shown in the Appendix A to this chapter.

Degrees of Freedom

When we earlier computed and defined standard deviation, it was presented as a descriptive statistic which was the square root of variance, i.e. the square root of the average squared deviation from the mean. (Recall that variance is equal to the sum of squared deviation divided by the number of observations.) When this particular definition is used descriptively only, it performs satisfactorily. When, however, it is carried over into sampling, and the sample variance is computed using it, then repetition of the calculation of sample variance over very many samples reveals that all the values obtained do not have the desirable property of averaging out to the population variance. The sample values are said to be 'biased'. To overcome this bias, sample variance is redefined as the sum of squared deviations divided by one less than the number of observations. This procedure results in values which do average out to the population variance. The sample standard deviation is, of course, the square root of the sample variance. The quantity in the denominator, which is one less than the number of observations, is the degrees of freedom and is used in preference to sample size.

The concept of degrees of freedom merits some explanation. Statistics that we can calculate from data take their properties from the variation present in the data—about which we have no control—and the number of independently varying quantities we include to obtain our statistic. Thus, if we take a sample of three items whose values are 17, 18 and 19, then the mean 18 is our calculated statistic and is obviously dependent on the fact that we have three quantities which generated it. If we had a sample of 39 items which generated the mean 18, then one would rightly expect the mean to have different (more desirable) statistical properties. In the case of the three values 17, 18, and 19, we say that the mean 18 is dependent on three degrees of freedom. That is, each of the three sample values is free to vary, giving three independently varying numbers to make up the mean.

Now consider the sample variance for our three sample members. The sample variance uses the deviations from the mean, which are -1, 0 and $+1$. Notice that these add to zero—an obvious feature of all deviations from a mean. Although the sample variance is based on these three deviations, only two of them are free to vary, say the -1 and the 0, because the third is the 'balancing item' necessary to make their sum zero. We have lost a degree of freedom, and this has come about by constraining our data to vary about the sample mean. We are using the sample mean as a pivot and balancing around it for our calculations. The resulting sample variance is based only on two degrees of freedom and takes its statistical properties accordingly. It is therefore preferable to define the sample variance as the sum of the squared deviations divided by the degrees of freedom (rather than by sample size).

The *t* Distribution

For testing hypotheses we calculate the difference between a sample value and the hypothesised value, and then standardise this difference by dividing by the standard error. The result of this—the test statistic—is then compared with a previously stated critical value such as 1·645 in our example above. The standard error used is calculated by taking the population standard deviation and dividing by the square root of sample size, and it should be the same whichever particular random sample we are using. However, the population standard deviation is not usually known, and so the sample standard deviation is used in its place. This latter does vary from sample to sample, and so into our test statistic has been introduced an extra source of sampling variation. The result is that we cannot expect our test statistic to have the same normal distribution with which it started, but rather to be more variable. This increased variability is reflected in the replacement of the 1·645, with which we compared, by a larger value, known as a '*t*' statistic. Instead of using values associated with the normal distribution, we replace them with larger values from the *t* distribution. It has already been mentioned in Chapter 5 that a requirement before we can safely use the *t* tables is that the original population is normally distributed, at least approximately.

Reference to a *t* table shows that it is in fact a series of tables, and very crudely speaking, there is a *t* table for every sample size (see Appendix 3b). Instead of sample size appears the phrase 'degrees of freedom'. There is a different line for each level of the degrees of freedom and, in effect, a different *t* table for every value of the degrees of freedom.

In the present example, namely testing the mean weight gain in a sample of babies, the degrees of freedom is one less than sample size, but there are times in more advanced work when it varies from this. Our sample of 32 babies produces a test statistic with 31 degrees of freedom, and it will be found on consulting a *t* table that the values in it are almost identical with the *z* values that would otherwise have been used. For samples of 30 or more items, it is sufficient to use *z* values and not make the switch to *t* values.

Let us say that our sample had consisted of 17 babies, with sample mean weight gain 203 g per week, and sample standard deviation 67·4. The standard error of the mean is approximately $67{\cdot}4 \div \sqrt{17} = 16{\cdot}35$, and the test statistic is $(203 - 170) \div 16{\cdot}35 = 2{\cdot}02$. The critical *t* value from tables has $17 - 1 = 16$ degrees of freedom, and we look up the *t* value which is exceeded by 5% of values. This is 1·746. The *z* value of 1·645 appears at the foot of the column containing 1·746, indicating that for large samples (above 30) where we need not use t, the z value coincides with the t value. Our test statistic 2·02 exceeds 1·746, and hence we say that we reject the null hypothesis at the 5% level (i.e. $P < 0{\cdot}05$).

The design of experiments is of major importance in clinical medicine. The following example is a simple one, and is intended to convey the basic concept of design, which itself is discussed more fully in Chapter 7, and utilises a simple t test.

A Matched Pair Example

If two treatments are under comparison, e.g. analgesics A and B, then clearly they must be used in circumstances where as much uncontrolled variation as possible is eliminated, so that any differences in performance can be attributed entirely to the analgesics. If two analgesics are used at different points in time on a particular patient, then as long as the patient's condition and circumstances are constant, he acts as his own 'control', and the difference in hours of relief from pain can be attributed to the difference in the effectiveness of the treatment. Suppose six patients exhibit the data shown in Table 7. The difference is computed for each patient as in the final column, and their mean is 0·1167, with standard deviation 0·2787. The formal procedure is as follows: We set up a null hypothesis, which postulates that the mean difference is zero, and an alternative hypothesis that the mean difference is positive (i.e. B provides more hours of relief than A).

Table 7

A Matched Pair (or Paired Difference) Example

Patient	Hours of Relief with A	Hours of Relief with B	Difference
A	2·7	3·1	0·4
B	2·9	3·3	0·4
C	4·1	3·8	−0·3
D	3·7	3·9	0·2
E	2·8	2·9	0·1
F	3·4	3·3	−0·1

The central limit theorem informs us that the sample mean difference will be distributed around the true value, with standard error calculated as the population standard deviation divided by the square root of sample size. The standard deviation is unknown, so we estimate it using the sample standard deviation to obtain

$$\frac{0{\cdot}2787}{\sqrt{6}} = 0{\cdot}1137$$

Since we have six observations, we retain five degrees of freedom when we use the sample standard deviation.

We now set acceptance and rejection regions, bearing in mind that the sample is small and the sample standard deviation is being used to estimate population standard deviation. As long as the population of differences can be assumed to be normally distributed, the t distribution operates. The significance level of 0·1 reveals that, with five degrees of freedom, the critical 't' value is 4·032. The sample value is 0·1167 and has a 't' value $(0{\cdot}1167-0)/0{\cdot}1137=1{\cdot}026$. Clearly the sample value lies within the acceptance region and there is no evidence to reject the null hypothesis of equality of performance of the analgesics.

The Chi-square Test

The chi-square test in its most popular and useful form enables us to check whether the rows are independent of the columns in a cross-tabulation of frequencies.

For example, suppose we have in Table 8 the data from an experiment to test whether three types of surface result in differing incidences of decubiti in elderly orthopaedic patients.

Table 8

Cross-tabulation of Incidence of Decubiti by Surface

Frequency (Number of Patients)	Surface A Low Air Loss Bed	Surface B Water Bed	Surface C Ripple Mattress
Decubiti observed	7	13	25
No decubiti observed	49	58	47

Testing the independence of the rows and columns means testing whether the surface is related to the incidence of decubiti. Table 8 which enumerates the patients in each category is called a 'contingency table', and the chi-square test indicates whether or not the distribution of the observed decubiti over the users of the different surfaces is 'even', or is apparently related to the type of surface.

The chi-squared test differs in nature from previous tests because it deals with differences between categories, in situations where precise quantitative measurement may not be possible. Thus, if alternative treatments are available, each of which can produce results categorised as, for example, full recovery, partial recovery, or no recovery, then the enumeration of the cases in each category provides the basis for the test. One would not deal with a 'measurement' of recovery beyond its classification, according to the pre-defined classes.

Suppose two treatment regimes are applied each to 100 patients, with the number of patients in each category as in Table 9.

Table 9

Results of Treating 200 Patients

Number of Patients	Some Success	No Success	Total
Treatment A	85	15	100
Treatment B	75	25	100
Total	160	40	200

Even if the treatments are, in the long term when applied to many patients, of equal value, when a single sample of 200 is used, some differences in success rates are inevitable. The chi-squared test checks whether this observed deviation is within the usual expected sampling range of variation. If the treatments were equal, Table 10 would have been obtained.

The figures in Table 10 are referred to as expected values. The individual deviations are given in Table 11.

The total 'algebraic' error is zero and, as usual in statistics, these deviations are squared to give Table 12.

Table 10

Results of Treating 200 Patients if Two Treatments of Equal Value

Number of Patients	Some Success	No Success	Total
Treatment A	80	20	100
Treatment B	80	20	100
Total	160	40	200

Finally, to obtain a 'total' of 'error' some sort of addition is required. However, arbitrary increases in the figures due to larger numbers being involved can occur. This is overcome by linking each 'deviation squared' to the expected value, which is a form of standardisation, and we obtain a 'relative' deviation, as in Table 13.

The total 'deviation' is the sum of the values in Table 13, i.e.

$$\frac{25}{80}+\frac{25}{80}+\frac{25}{20}+\frac{25}{20} = 3{\cdot}125$$

The tabulated values of chi-squared are now consulted. These provide the upper limits that could occur in random sampling of the statistic we have calculated under the null hypothesis of equality.

Given 100 people in each treatment (160 successes and 40 fails), the numbers within the table have very little freedom to distribute themselves. Thus, if we know that there are 85 people of group A on whom there has been some success, by appropriate subtractions,

Table 11

Deviations from Expected Numbers

+5	−5
−5	+5

Table 12

Squared Deviations from Expected Numbers

25	25
25	25

Table 13

Squared Deviations Divided by Expected Values

25/80	25/20
25/80	25/20

all the other values in the table have no freedom to vary. We say there is one degree of freedom, and this is used when consulting the chi-squared table in Appendix 3. We obtain:

$$\text{chi-squared}\ {}^{0{\cdot}05}_{1\ \text{df}} = 3{\cdot}841$$

This is the value above which 5% of values would be legitimately expected to fall. We call this our 'rejection region'. It can be seen that our 'test statistic' does not fall here and we cannot reject the null hypothesis of equality. Thus, on the face of a casual inspection, treatment A is better, but there is no statistical evidence at the 5% level to suggest any real difference between the treatments. We would say that there is no statistically significant difference ($P = 0{\cdot}05$).

The rule for expected values is as follows. For any cell in row r, column k, the expected value is

$$\frac{\text{Row r total} \times \text{Column k total}}{\text{Grand total}}$$

and the degrees of freedom is

$$(\text{Number of rows} - 1) \times (\text{Number of columns} - 1)$$

We can easily extend the chi-squared test to consider several rows and columns simultaneously. For example, Table 14 shows a 2 × 3 table for 952 children seen in an asthma clinic. They are grouped into 209 for whom environmental factors were believed not to be associated with the onset of asthma, and 743 where environmental factors clearly were relevant. The degree of severity of the asthma attack was either mild, moderate, or severe.

The chi-squared test tells us whether the figures displayed in the

Table 14

Contingency Table for 952 Patients, Showing Severity of Asthma and Presence or Absence of Environmental Factors

	Degree of Severity			
	Mild	Moderate	Severe	Totals
No environmental factors present	158	35	16	209
Environmental factors present	450	160	133	743
Totals	608	195	149	952

table differ significantly from those which could occur by chance on the assumption of the null hypothesis that degree of severity is unrelated to environmental factors.

Table 15 shows the values that would be expected if the null hypothesis were true. These can be obtained using the formula given above, or by the following method. For all the 952 patients irrespective of whether there were or were not environmental associations, a proportion (608/952) had a mild attack. Hence, if environment is irrelevant to severity, then this proportion should apply to the 209 with no environmental factors, as well as the 743 with environmental factors. For the former group it should produce $608/952 \times 209 = 133{\cdot}48$ patients who are in the 'no environmental factors' group and have a mild attack. The actual number from Table 14 is of course 158, and we are concerned as to whether the discrepancy could be due to pure chance. Working out all the expected values in the above manner produces Table 15.

Table 15

Numbers of Patients 'Expected' in Each Category if Environmental Factors are Unrelated to Severity of Asthma

	Degree of Severity		
	Mild	Moderate	Severe
No environmental factors present	133·48	42·81	32·71
Environmental factors present	474·52	152·19	116·29

The calculated chi-squared statistic is

$$(158-133{\cdot}48)^2/133{\cdot}48+(35-42{\cdot}81)^2/42{\cdot}81+$$
$$(16-32{\cdot}71)^2/32{\cdot}71+(450-474{\cdot}52)^2/474{\cdot}52+$$
$$(160-152{\cdot}19)^2/152{\cdot}19+(133-116{\cdot}29)^2/116{\cdot}29 = 18{\cdot}56$$

There are 2 degrees of freedom. From the chi-square table the probability that pure chance will generate a value above 10·6 is 0·005. We say that our results are significant, with $P<0{\cdot}005$ because our value of 18·56 is so much above the values likely to occur by chance. In other words, the results of our survey suggest very strongly that asthmatic severity and the presence of environmental factors in the diagnosis are related.

The chi-squared test is very widely used, but is non-specific. We did not test above whether severity was greater or less in a specific group—only whether a difference overall existed. The type of data with which the chi-squared deals is enumerative—i.e. obtained by counting—and does not need to be amenable to detailed measurement, merely categorisation. The test works best when the expected values in each position of the table are at least 5. When this is not so, judicious merging of rows and/or columns is desirable to build up to 5. The merging should only be done in a meaningful manner. In our above example, it might be reasonable, if we were dealing with smaller numbers, to merge 'mild' with 'moderate', or 'moderate' with 'severe', depending on our focus of attention. It would probably be irrelevant to merge mild with severe—the result would have no meaning. Although the data in the chi-squared test needs to be enumerative, in effect the test checks whether a set of two or more proportions differ significantly.

Non-parametric Tests

Earlier in this chapter we concentrated on testing hypotheses about parameters such as the mean, or a proportion with a particular characteristic. When dealing with small sample means we needed to assume that the population values are normally distributed.

Statistical tests which are concerned with characteristics of groups but not specifically with parameters and/or do not require strict assumptions concerning the distribution of the underlying population are referred to as non-parametric tests. The chi-squared test with its interest in whether there are general differences between categories in a contingency table may be considered in the class of non-parametric tests.

Non-parametric methods are frequently used in situations where the data consists of observations which are in rank order. Many practical research problems require subjective ratings on a numerical scale. If a doctor rates patient A's condition as 4, and that of patient B as 2 on a scale of 1 to 7, where 7 is perfectly well, these numbers do not have full 'mathematical' significance, even though they do serve a useful medical purpose. A is not twice as healthy as B. If we have a patient C who is rated 6, he is not three times as healthy as B, nor could we even say that the health difference between A and B is the same as that between A and C. Neither ratios between values, nor intervals between them mean anything. All that is being said by the numbers is that C is healthier than A, who in turn is healthier than B. The individuals are thus given a rank, or order, and we say that the scale of measurement has only ordinal significance, and is not amenable to ordinary arithmetic. We could just as well have given A a value of 74, B a value 76 and C a value 1947. Statistical tests on means, variances and standard deviations are not appropriate or valid for this kind of data.

Sometimes even ordinal measurement on some sort of scale is either impossible or not necessary. We can compare data where the 'scale' consists of two points only: 'better' and 'worse'.

The result of using ranks as our values and not the original measurements, or of using criteria such as 'better' or 'worse' is that the resulting non-parametric tests do waste some information and are often not as 'sharp' as parametric tests. On the other hand, when the raw data has doubtful precision, or is only subjectively estimated or judged, then ranking may be a more acceptable process than handling the raw data, and the tests needed would be non-parametric.

People who use non-parametric tests are usually comfortable with them because they do not read too much into the data, and because they do not run the risk of violating assumptions on which parametric tests such as '*t*' rest.

Four non-parametric tests which have wide usage are the sign test, the Wilcoxon signed rank test, the Mann-Whitney U test, and the Wilcoxon rank sum test. Examples of these follow.

The Sign Test

The sign test is one of the simplest non-parametric tests to use. Observations are collected in pairs, and we record whether the difference in each pair is negative, zero or positive. To illustrate this, suppose that on 10 randomly chosen patients we evaluate treatment 1, and on 10 other patients, matched person by person carefully with our first 10, we evaluate another treatment (treatment 2). The patients are listed in Table 16, and the numbering and lettering indicates that, for example, B_1 receives treatment 1, and has been carefully matched with patient B_2 who receives treatment 2. Suppose it is judged that A_1 does better than A_2. However we score them A_1 has a higher score than A_2, so the difference $A_1 - A_2$ is positive. Suppose B_1 does less well than B_2. Then, however we score $B_1 - B_2$ as negative. The plus and minus signs obtained for the 10 matched pairs are shown in Table 16. The two zeroes indicate equal outcomes, and are now subsequently ignored.

If the two treatments are equal we would expect roughly as many plus signs as minus signs. We have eight valid untied observations, of which five are minus signs. Thus, a proportion (5/8) are negative. The question we now have to resolve is this: under a hypothesis that plus and minus signs are equally likely, is it possible and reasonably easy in a sampling situation with eight results to find five pluses and three minuses? Intuitively, one might expect that this would be easy to find, and the exact probability of *at least* 5/8 of the signs being negative can be worked out to be 0·36 (using the Binomial distribution referred to in Appendix 2). It seems, therefore, that the sampling result is quite typical of what could occur if the treatments are of equal value, and so there are no strong reasons presented to reject the hypothesis of equality of the

Table 16

The Sign Test: Information on Differences Between Matched Pairs of Patients

Treatment 1	A_1	B_1	C_1	D_1	E_1	F_1	G_1	H_1	I_1	J_1
Treatment 2	A_2	B_2	C_2	D_2	E_2	F_2	G_2	H_2	I_2	J_2
Difference	+	−	0	+	−	−	−	0	+	−

treatments. If we had started out to check whether treatment 2 was better than treatment 1, then we should indeed be looking for mostly minus signs in our results. With a significance level, P, at 0·05, to reject the null hypothesis of equality the sample proportion would have needed to fall much further into the upper tail of the distribution than it actually has.

It should be noticed that no assumptions have been necessary about the distribution of scores in either group. We do not even need 'measures' of treatment effectiveness, only a judgement of which is better, or whether the treatments are equal.

To take another example of the sign test, this time using actual rankings on a scale, suppose that a patient satisfaction study is being carried out, and patients are asked to rate on a scale 1 to 5 their general comfort at night, and again during the day. A score of 5 indicates total satisfaction with comfort, whilst 1 indicates maximum dissatisfaction. The results are shown in Table 17.

We now use the signs of the differences to indicate whether the patients really show a difference between night comfort and day comfort. Zeroes are excluded, because they indicate a tie. We have 21 plus signs and 8 minus signs. Intuitively, it looks as though night comfort usually beats day comfort. If the two were equal, we would expect about equal numbers of plus and minus signs. That is, the proportion of plus signs should be 1/2. No sample would be expected to generate a value exactly at 1/2. The question to decide is when is the departure from 1/2 so great that we begin to feel quite strongly that 1/2 is not the true underlying value. Formally, we set up the null hypothesis that the two comfort levels are the same and thus the proportion of plus signs is 1/2. The alternative hypothesis depends on whether anything has been asserted about the relative comfort levels. The alternative would reflect the assertion. Let us suppose that we are testing as the alternative hypothesis that night and day comfort differ, but not in any particular direction. This sort of test is a two tail test. The test is on our observed proportion of plus signs, namely 21/29†, and gives the result that at the 5% level, there is a significant difference between night and day comfort. The result is saying that when night care and day care are equal for the population of patients, a random sample of 21/29 plus signs is extremely unlikely, purely by chance ($P < 0{\cdot}05$),

† The test can be carried out using the probabilities from the Binomial distribution, or the approximate probabilities from the normal distribution as an approximation.

Table 17

The Sign Test: Information on Differences Relating to the Same Patient

Patients	Night Rating = A	Day Rating = B	Sign of A − B
1	3	2	+
2	4	1	+
3	3	2	+
4	2	1	+
5	4	3	+
6	3	2	+
7	3	3	0
8	5	4	+
9	4	3	+
10	3	3	0
11	3	3	0
12	2	3	−
13	4	4	0
14	3	2	+
15	4	3	+
16	5	4	+
17	5	5	0
18	3	4	−
19	4	3	+
20	4	2	+
21	5	4	+
22	4	4	0
23	4	5	−
24	3	5	−
25	4	4	0
26	5	4	+
27	4	5	−
28	4	3	+
29	3	2	+
30	3	1	+
31	5	1	+
32	3	4	−
33	2	5	−
34	5	3	+
35	4	2	+
36	2	3	−

and hence the sample results show an apparently heavy preference for night care which is sufficient to reject our hypothesis of equality.

The Wilcoxon Signed Rank Test

The sign test we have just considered uses the signs of the differences between paired observations, such as individually matched patients, or before and after data on the same patients, or data on 'related' patients such as husbands and wives. The Wilcoxon signed rank test requires as data not only the signs of the differences between pairs of observations, but also the relative ranking of those differences. From this information the test can determine whether, for example, before and after data on the same patient for a sample is obtained from identical distributions, or whether the 'after' situation differs from the 'before'. This test uses both rank sums and signs of paired differences, i.e. more information than the sign test, and in that sense is more efficient. On the other hand, there will be many occasions on which relative ranking of differences is not known, and the sign test will have to be performed if we are to decide whether our two related samples come from identical distributions.

As an example of the Wilcoxon signed rank test, suppose that in a sample of 15 people (Table 18), we have taken measurements on reaction time before and after drinking a double whisky. It will be assumed that the 15 people are matched in relevant variables such as age, sex, general health, occupation, drinking habits and so on. Our objective is to test whether there is a difference in reaction time due to the alcohol. If we could assume that the data came from normally distributed populations, then a parametric '*t*' test can be carried out on the differences between each person's before and after time. The objective would be to test whether the mean difference differs significantly from zero.

However, if normality is not reasonable to assume—perhaps because we have no experience of this type of data—then the non-parametric Wilcoxon signed rank test is appropriate. To carry out the test requires us to calculate the list of differences between before and after readings, and then, temporarily ignoring whether differences are plus or minus, to write by each difference its rank, which will be a number from 1 to 15, because we have 15 pairs of

Table 18

The Wilcoxon Signed Rank Test for Two Related Samples

Participants	A	B	C	D	E	F	G	H	I	J	K	L	M	N	O
Reaction time 'before'	2·0	4·7	6·2	7·3	4·6	5·3	5·5	6·1	7·3	4·7	5·1	3·9	2·8	3·1	4·0
Reaction time 'after'	4·1	7·3	6·1	8·9	6·5	7·2	5·4	6·0	9·4	6·3	4·8	4·1	3·0	3·0	4·0
Differences	−2·1	−2·6	0·1	−1·6	−1·9	−1·9	0·1	0·1	−2·1	−1·6	0·3	−0·2	−0·2	0·1	0

observations. The sum of the ranks of the positive differences and the sum of the ranks of the negative differences are calculated and, if the before and after readings do not differ, should be roughly equal. There is a simple formula to calculate what the mean of these two rank sums should be, so if either deviates considerably from the mean, this constitutes evidence to reject the hypothesis that before and after reaction times are the same.

The formula for the mean rank sum for n measurements is

$$0{\cdot}25\, n\, (n+1),$$

and the test carried out to see whether either of the obtained rank sums differ is a simple z test using the normal distribution, since sums of items, such as ranks, are normally distributed according to the 'Central Limit Theorem', described in Chapter 5. The actual conclusion in this case is to reject the null hypothesis at the 5% level of significance and conclude that there are differences in reaction times. The calculations are shown in Appendix B to this chapter.

The Wilcoxon signed rank test is quick and easy to perform provided the z test is first mastered. If a pair of observations tie, they are omitted, as with the sign test. Where ranks tie, both are given the same rank, which is the mean of the rank placings they occupy. Thus, if four observations rank equal fifth, they occupy places 5, 6, 7 and 8 and are given rank 6·5.

The Wilcoxon Rank Sum Test

A whole 'family' of non-parametric tests under the name 'rank sum' test exist, among the most well known being the Mann-Whitney U test and the Wilcoxon rank sum test. These tests enable us to determine whether two independent samples have been drawn from the same population, or from two different populations. The difference between, on the one hand, the Wilcoxon rank sum and Mann-Whitney U test and, on the other hand, the previously described sign test and Wilcoxon signed rank test is due to the fact that the latter two were carried out on related, or 'paired', samples, whereas the U test and the Wilcoxon rank sum test use unrelated samples. The Mann-Whitney U test is actually equivalent to the Wilcoxon rank sum test, and the two lead to identical conclusions. For simplicity we will describe the latter.

Let us suppose that we are considering psychiatric patients in two separate institutions to find out whether length of hospital stay differs between the institutions. If the two groups of patients are very similar in a number of relevant characteristics and thus can be considered to be matched (but not in pairs), then it would seem reasonable to attribute differences in stay to institutional factors. The fact that we may know that lengths of hospital stay are not normally distributed pushes us into a non-parametric testing situation, rather than a parametric procedure. Subjective measures would also require a non-parametric test because they have no real mathematical meaning beyond that which their ordinal significance conveys. For example, instead of comparing lengths of stay, we might be comparing patients on a disability index which rates 'well patients' as 1, and the most severely disabled as 10.

Let us suppose that in Table 19 we have randomly chosen 17 patients from hospital A, and 23 from hospital B, and that the groups are matched in general characteristics relevant to length of hospitalisation. We may wish to test whether the samples are taken from the same population, with the same mean or median.

We pool the 40 observations and put them into rank order from smallest to largest. The smallest is given rank 1, the next smallest rank 2 and so on. Once we have the rankings the samples are separated, and for each sample we find the sum of the ranks it contains. These rank sums, called W, are our test statistics.

The rationale of both the Mann-Whitney U test and the Wilcoxon rank sum test centres on the idea that if the sum of the rankings for one group differs greatly from the sum of the rankings for the other group, then it is reasonable to conclude that there is a difference in the central locations of the groups.

Table 19

The Wilcoxon Rank Sum Test for Two Independent Samples

Hospital A—Length of stay in days											
1	0	3	5	4	14	12	14	13			
16	18	5	11	14	15	12	12				
Hospital B—Length of stay in days											
32	29	19	17	21	26	22	17	7	2	28	22
6	17	23	39	41	48	26	34	33	32	10	

High ranks for members of group A would indicate a situation where A values are typically bigger than B values, showing greater lengths of stay in hospital A, and we would see a large value for the A rank-sum. If there is no difference between hospitals A and B, then the A observations and the B observations should be randomly scattered in a similar manner over the rankings from 1 to 40.

The W statistic has been constructed as a sum of a set of values, and it therefore has a normal distribution. We can use the z test to see whether W for A differs significantly from the mean value we would expect, which is given by the simple formula

$$0{\cdot}5\, n_{\mathrm{A}}\, (n_{\mathrm{A}} + n_{\mathrm{B}} + 1)$$

where n_{A} and n_{B} are the sample sizes in groups A and B, respectively. (The sample B rank sum is automatically determined by the sample A rank sum, because the total of both rank sums is fixed by the number of observations. Hence, we need look only at the sample A rank sum.) The appendix to this chapter shows the calculation procedure, and the results in this case are that we should reject the hypothesis that the lengths of stay at A and B are the same, at the 5% significance level. We have evidence which suggests that stay lengths differ.

The example we have used is considerably simplified and contained only a few tied observations. Where there are many ties, or for situations where sample sizes are smaller than those in our example, then alternative methods are available. The detailed techniques of non-parametric statistics can fill a complete book by themselves. We have described only four simplified tests.

All four of these non-parametric tests have this in common: they change the analysis from whatever original units were used to the analysis of a simple variable, typically a sum, whose distribution is easily handled and well known. There are very many non-parametric tests available to suit differing situations, and the four chosen for presentation here have been selected partly because of their importance in recent medical work which uses subjective measurement scales, or small samples from non-normal populations, and partly to convey the flavour of non-parametric testing.

Appendix A—A Test on a Proportion

Suppose we wish to test the proposition that 70% of people who display symptom A also have associated symptom B. We start with a null hypothesis which states that we expect the proportion to be 0·7. Should we reject 0·7 we need to specify in advance of sampling an alternative hypothesis, and let us take the alternative to be that the proportion is not equal to 0·7.

A random sample of 49 people is surveyed, and 40 display symptoms A and B, which represents a proportion 40/49 = 0·82. Is this evidence consistent with our hypothesis of 0·7, or does it offer a strong suggestion that 0·7 is in error? The answer lies in knowing the distribution of sample proportions that could occur when the population proportion is 0·7. This distribution is closely approximated by a normal distribution with a standard deviation known as 'the standard error of the proportion' given by the formula:

$$\sqrt{\frac{(\text{Proportion}) \times (1 - \text{Proportion})}{\text{Sample size}}}$$

The standard error thus would be expected to be

$$\sqrt{\frac{(0{\cdot}7)(0{\cdot}3)}{49}} = 0{\cdot}065$$

In this situation we are dealing with a two-tailed test, meaning that we are prepared to reject the value 0·7 if the sample proportion is either significantly less than or significantly more than 0·7. If we set our significance level P at 0·05, we would reject the hypothesis of 0·7 if the sample value falls either in the lowest 0·025 (2·5%) or the highest 0·025 of the possible distribution around 0·7. The 'z' values at the two critical points which determine where these regions start are obtained as $-1{\cdot}96$ and $+1{\cdot}96$ from the table of the standard normal distribution. We then compare the z value of the sample statistic 0·7 with these two critical values. Recall that z is the number of standard deviations that out point lies away from the midpoint of the distribution. Therefore:

$$\begin{aligned} z &= (\text{Sample value} - \text{Distribution mean})/\text{Standard error of sample value} \\ &= (0{\cdot}82 - 0{\cdot}7)/0{\cdot}065 \\ &= 1{\cdot}85 \end{aligned}$$

Since 1·85 is less than 1·96 we conclude that the sample proportion observed does not conflict with the null hypothesis of 0·7, and we have no evidence to reject 0·7 at the 5% level ($P = 0{\cdot}05$).

Appendix B—The Wilcoxon Signed Rank Test for Two Related Samples

Participants	A	B	C	D	E	F	G	H	I	J	K	L	M	N	O
Reaction time 'before'	2·0	4·7	6·2	7·3	4·6	5·3	5·5	6·1	7·3	4·7	5·1	3·9	2·8	3·1	4·0
Reaction time 'after'	4·1	7·3	6·1	8·9	6·5	7·2	5·4	6·0	9·4	6·3	4·8	4·1	3·0	3·0	4·0
Differences	−2·1	−2·6	0·1	−1·6	−1·9	−1·9	0·1	0·1	−2·1	−1·6	0·3	−0·2	−0·2	0·1	0

For the untied observations only:

Positive Differences	Actual Ranks		Ranks Given
0·1	1	=	2·5
0·1	1	=	2·5
0·1	1	=	2·5
0·1	1	=	2·5
0·3	7	=	7

Sum of ranks given for positive differences = 17

Negative Differences	Actual Ranks		Ranks Given
−2·1	12	=	12·5
−2·6	14	=	14
−1·6	8	=	8·5
−1·9	10	=	10·5
−1·9	10	=	10·5
−2·1	12	=	12·5
−1·6	8	=	8·5
−0·2	5	=	5·5
−0·2	5	=	5·5

Sum of ranks given for negative differences = 88

We test whether 17 (or 88) differs significantly from $0{\cdot}25\ n\ (n+1) = 0{\cdot}25 \times 14 \times 15 = 52{\cdot}5$, which is the mean of the rank sums.

The variance of the rank sums is $n\ (n+1)(2n+1)/24 = 14(15)(29)/24 = 253{\cdot}75$ and so the standard deviation is 15·93 (i.e. the square root of the variance).

The z statistic is $(17 - 52{\cdot}5)/15{\cdot}93 = -2{\cdot}23$, which numerically exceeds $-1{\cdot}96$, and is a statistically significant result, $P < 0{\cdot}05$.

N.B. Where there are equal ranks, as above where four differences are equal first in rank, the 'Rank Given' is the mean of the ranks which would have been obtained if the values had been unequal and ranked 1, 2, 3 and 4, namely 2·5.

Appendix C—The Wilcoxon Rank Sum Test for Two Independent Samples

Hospital A—Length of stay in days

1	0	3	5	4	14	12	14	13
16	18	5	11	14	15	12	12	

Hospital B—Length of stay in days

32	29	19	17	21	26	22	17	7	2	28	22
6	17	23	39	41	48	26	34	33	32	10	

Data for Wilcoxon Rank Sum Test:

		Pooled Ranks				Pooled Ranks	
Ordered Data	**Hospital**	**A**	**B**	**Ordered Data**	**Hospital**	**A**	**B**
0	A	1		11	A	11	
1	A	2		12	A	13	
2	B		3	12	A	13	
3	A	4		12	A	13	
4	A	5		13	A	15	
5	A	6·5		14	A	17	
5	A	6·5		14	A	17	
6	B		8	14	A	17	
7	B		9	15	A	19	
10	B		10	16	A	20	

17	B		22	26	B		30·5
17	B		22	28	B		32
17	B		22	29	B		33
18	A	24		32	B		34·5
19	B		25	32	B		34·5
21	B		26	33	B		36
22	B		27·5	34	B		37
22	B		27·5	39	B		38
23	B		29	41	B		39
26	B		30·5	48	B		40

Sum of ranks for A = 204
Sum of ranks for B = 616

The mean rank sum for A is $n_A\,(n_A+n_B+1)/2$. In this case the mean is $17\times 41/2=348{\cdot}5$. The variance of the rank sums for A is $n_A n_B\,(n_A+n_B+1)/12=17\times 23\times 41/12=1335{\cdot}9167$.

The z statistic is calculated as

$$\frac{\text{Actual rank sum}-\text{Mean of rank sum}}{\text{Standard deviation of rank sum}}=\frac{W-\dfrac{n_A\,(n_A+n_B+1)}{2}}{\sqrt{\dfrac{n_A n_B\,(n_A+n_B+1)}{12}}}=\frac{204-348{\cdot}5}{36{\cdot}55}$$

and in this case is $-3{\cdot}95$. The critical z values are $\pm 1{\cdot}96$, and since $-3{\cdot}95$ is numerically greater than $-1{\cdot}96$, we reject the null hypothesis at the 5% level (i.e. $P<0{\cdot}05$).

7

Clinical Trials and the Design of Experiments

Introduction

New drugs and new treatments require scientific testing prior to general usage. The standard method of testing is the clinical trial. The results of such a trial are usually expressed probabilistically, and 'significant' differences between a 'control group' and a 'trial group' are sought. The control group receive either a placebo, or a 'traditional' or existing treatment, whilst the 'trial' group receive the new drug or treatment. The design of the clinical trial is crucial to the validity of the subsequent results and should always be made in close association with a statistician and, if relevant, a computer analyst.

Clinical trials of new drugs or treatments have, in general, as essential pre-requisites, clearly stated objectives, defined criteria for evaluation of outcome, good design and plan for analysis, a suitable 'control' group, and an agreement on the medical ethics of the trial.

The control group should consist of patients matched in characteristics to the treatment group, and ideally patients should be allocated to one group or the other in a random or mechanical way which precludes the intervention of judgement about who is most suited to each group. The characteristics of members of each group need clear advance definition so that exclusion of complicated or unusually complex conditions may be made.

A placebo should normally be used for the control group when there is no conventional treatment available.

In the most desirable experiment neither the doctor nor the patient knows which patient receives the new treatment and which the orthodox or placebo. This sort of trial is known as 'double-blind', and may require extra medical assistance to monitor other medical factors and make assessments and evaluations from specimen analysis and appropriate tests.

Difficulties often exist with control groups which can make them unsatisfactory, and so important checks need to be made on them. For example, information may be available on certain responses in patients from historically available data prior to the introduction of the new treatment. If the existing information is to be used as though previous patients are the control group, and then the new treatment is to be given to an experimental group we must be completely satisfied that previous patients are comparable in the important variables such as age, sex, primary diagnosis, secondary diagnosis, etc. We also need to be satisfied that the other factors relevant to outcome, such as nursing policies and staffing levels, weather conditions, and other morbidity factors have not changed. In short, detailed record analysis of previous patients has to be undertaken, and such records may be inadequate or unavailable.

Comparability problems can bedevil trials which involve comparisons between patients in different hospitals in much the same way. The other 'uncontrolled' factors can be intervening in the results to an unknown extent. Thus, differences ascribed by researchers to the treatment may be due to paramedical or non-medical differences which were uncontrolled. Where volunteers are used for a treatment the selection of a control group who are matched may present difficulties. When patients are given the opportunity to participate or not, differential responses by certain types of patient may cause bias.

The problems of valid control groups which match treatment groups in as many characteristics as possible frequently receives inadequate attention in medical research because of various difficulties, expense and time. It is fairly rare that total absence of 'controls' is acceptable. This would occur where a particular outcome is universal in a specific diagnosis. Any reversal of this may be so dramatic as not to require controls.

With patients who have a relatively stable chronic condition it may be possible to use the patient as his own control. The patient has alternative treatments separated by sufficient time for the effect of the previous treatment to disappear, but short enough to ensure no real change in the patient's condition. This sort of trial is known as a 'cross-over' trial. With conditions which are progressive, cross-over trials are not practicable. The trial of two analgesics in this manner is shown in Chapter 6, where the analysis is carried out.

Sometimes patients may be matched in pairs, so that each pair is very similar in the factors such as age, sex, disease, condition and so on. On a random basis one of the pair receives the treatment under test, the other either the orthodox treatment or a placebo. As with the cross-over trial, the analysis for matched pairs is fairly simple and lends itself to a technique known as sequential analysis, which will be discussed shortly.

Experimental Designs

Experimental design usually refers to the statistical construction and plan for analysis involved when the comparison of treatments, etc., is the objective.

Experiments to test new treatments are expensive. Many experiments have been conducted without specific thought—in advance—about the objectives, hypotheses and methods of analysis, resulting in a frustrating visit to a statistician who says that very little can be inferred from the results, and some important questions cannot be answered.

Experiments need careful design both to eliminate as much uncontrollable variation as possible and to maximise the precision of the results relative to the costs.

There exist a multitude of possible designs and doctors considering a 'trial' of any kind are well advised to consult a statistician far in advance of any plan to experiment. The actual design and analysis are best carried out by a professional statistical adviser, but nevertheless some of the main types of design available will be described in general terms.

In Chapter 6 the simplest kind of experiment is described, where patients act as their own control and each try two analgesics. The analysis required is the 't' test on the mean difference in hours of pain relief, obtained by getting the individual differences for each patient, and then averaging. Use of the t test requires that the differences come from a normally distributed population (otherwise a non-parametric test as discussed in Chapter 6, such as the Wilcoxon signed rank test may be used). This sort of trial, it will be recalled, is referred to as a cross-over trial.

To take another example using a cross-over design, suppose we are testing the effectiveness of a new drug for asthma. It is administered to individual patients who are then asked to exercise, so that the severity of the asthmatic attack induced can be measured. Since each test subject is almost certain to experience an asthmatic attack, few patients will volunteer so typically a small sample will result.

Each patient performs the exercises twice. The first time, the new drug—which we may call 'Easy Air'—is used to reduce the severity. After a lapse of time sufficient to ensure that the asthmatic response to new exercise is unconnected to that of the first exercise, the experiment is repeated with the orthodox treatment (or a placebo) which we may call 'Orth Air'. The patient is thus his own 'control' in that all other factors relevant to asthma are the same at each trial (i.e. under control) and so any difference observed in the response can be attributed to the difference in the drugs.

The asthmatic response to the exercise should be measured in a way that is both valid and reliable, and we may call the measure obtained the Asthma Score. Suppose that this runs from zero (i.e. no attack of any kind) to 100, which represents a very severe attack judged by pre-defined and agreed criteria. Table 20 shows the results from a sample of 12 patients.

We are interested in the difference between the drugs and column 4 of Table 20 records this for each patient. It is immediately obvious that the Easy Air score is usually lower, and we measure the sample mean difference score as 11·33, with a standard deviation of 11·23. We now have to decide whether, under a null hypothesis that the treatments are of equal value, a score for the mean difference of 11·33 is typical of those that could occur by chance. The appropriate test for this design is the t test, and when t is calculated it is $-3{\cdot}5$. On consulting a t table we find that there is a probability of less than 0·01 of obtaining a sample t value of $-3{\cdot}5$ if the scores are really equal in the population. Accordingly the hypothesis of no difference in severity is rejected in favour of one of a difference in severity. If the asthma attack severity was subjectively assessed and was not a physical reproducible measure then, as in the previous example, we should prefer a non-parametric test. In this case the Wilcoxon signed rank test as described in Chapter 6 would be appropriate.

A similar analysis can take place where patients are matched in pairs. The difference between the members of each pair is recorded,

Table 20

Scores in a Cross-over Trial Using the Patient as his own 'Control' and Resulting in a Paired Difference Test

Patient	Score Using Easy Air	Score Using Orth Air	Difference (col. 3 – col. 2)
A	17	24	7
B	23	24	1
C	37	45	8
D	29	29	0
E	31	48	17
F	22	61	39
G	15	28	13
H	29	26	–3
I	25	41	16
J	20	27	7
K	13	33	20
L	17	28	11

and from it the mean difference between treatments can be calculated.

At the next 'level' of experiment we may, for example, be dealing with two groups of patients who are not matched in pairs but who, over the whole of each group, are broadly similar in important medical characteristics relevant to the outcome of their treatment. One group receives the orthodox regime (or a placebo) and the other the new treatment, and we analyse to see if the typical outcomes for each group differ. Outcome of course must be defined in advance as for example a parameter such as mean time to reach a certain condition, or proportion of patients manifesting certain characteristics.

To illustrate the use of two matched groups suppose that, as a result of delays between the first part of the trial (using Easy Air) and the second, that some patients are no longer available and consequently instead of using the patients as their own control, it is necessary to take a matched group for the Orth Air trial. In this case the groups need to be as similar as possible in as many relevant factors as possible, so that the only differences relate to which treatment is used. Table 21 shows the results, and it will be noticed that the groups are not equal in size and that the

Table 21

Score in a Trial Using Two Matched Groups, and Resulting in a Test of the Difference Between Two Means

Group 1 Using Easy Air	Group 2 Using Orth Air
17	86
23	20
37	40
29	65
31	38
22	41
15	19
29	39
25	57
20	29
13	48
17	

observations are not 'paired'; so we cannot look at individual differences. Instead we have a less powerful test than before to help us. We calculate the mean and standard deviation for each group. For the Easy Air group the mean asthma score is 23·17, with standard deviation 7·27. For the Orth Air group the mean asthma score is higher, as might be expected, at 43·82, with standard deviation 19·75. The question then arises as to whether this observed lower mean score with the new drug could be due to chance, or whether it is indicative of a preferable treatment. Formally we take a null hypothesis which says that the difference between the mean scores is zero (i.e. nullify the claim to Easy Air being better than Orth Air) and consider whether the observed difference of 20·65 could be due to chance. In this case we find the t statistic to be $-3{\cdot}71$, which numerically exceeds the tabulated t at the 1% level. We conclude that we should reject the hypothesis at the 1% level of significance. If it is agreed that asthma scores are subjective, then we should have used, for example, the Mann-Whitney U test or the Wilcoxon rank sum test.

It is when we are comparing three or more treatments that the technique known as analysis of variance is required. Depending on the complexity of factors in the experiment several 'models' are common.

The most common technique for multiple simultaneous comparison is a completely randomised design in which patients are randomly assigned to a group, and then measurements are made on the individuals in each group. A mean can be obtained for each group, and if the treatments are of equal value, the variation displayed between these means should not differ markedly from the variation to be found *within* the groups. If, on the other hand, the treatments are producing on average real differences so that the means are quite widely separated, then the variation between them will be significantly greater than the variation to be found within the groups. The technique of analysis of variance provides a formal test to see whether the group means really differ.

As an example of the technique of analysis of variance with three or more matched groups, consider a three-way comparison between Easy Air, Orth Air and a placebo. In this case we are looking for any general differences that may result, without being specific about a particular pair. Table 22 shows the results when the placebo group, who do the same exercises and are matched to the other groups, are included.

It is noticeable from Table 22 that the groups are now smaller. This can easily happen because the constraints of matching cause

Table 22

Score in a Trial Using Three Matched Groups and Resulting in an Analysis of Variance to Test for Differences Between the Groups

Group 1 Using Easy Air	Group 2 Using Orth Air	Group 3 Using a Placebo
17	86	51
23	20	37
37	40	93
29	65	49
31	38	88
22	41	86
15	19	59
29	39	65
25	57	49

some patients to be eliminated. It is not essential to make the groups equal, but the calculations are a little simpler.

The analysis of variance—despite its name—actually compares the three group means. We set off with a null hypothesis of equality between the means, and we test this by analysing two relevant variances. The first is the variance of the members within each group. The second is the variance between the means of the three groups. The total variance we observe over all the patients in all the groups is made up of the variance existing within each group together with the variance between the groups. If the groups really do not differ, then the variation between them should be much the same as the variation within them. By obtaining the ratio of these two variances and observing whether the ratio differs from unity by an amount beyond that likely due to chance, we can establish whether a difference does appear to exist. If it does we would conclude that the three 'treatments' really do produce different results. In our example, the statistical test results in the ratio of variances (called 'F') being 11·1 which, after consulting the appropriate table (usually known as an F table), tells us that there is some evidence of a real difference ($P < 0{\cdot}01$). The F tests assume normally distributed populations. Where no such assumption is reasonable the non-parametric analogy to the one-way analysis of variance is the Kruskal-Wallis analysis of variance.

The completely randomised design such as that for Easy Air, Orth Air and the placebo is simple, obvious and unsophisticated. Any number of treatments can be compared, and it is not necessary to have equal numbers in each group. Consequently, 'missing' observations (due to, say, a failure to record or an exclusion of the patient during the trial due to other factors) are not a problem.

Where the patients themselves display clear blocks in each grouping which would be expected to cause difference in their response to treatment, then these specific 'block' effects would be lost with a completely randomised design, as just described. A simple example would be where we have three treatments applied to patients whose age groups range from 15–24 through to 85–94. It would clearly be worth recognising the age variation by specifically structuring the experiment for it. Not to do so would weaken the results, because the age (or 'block') effect would, in a completely randomised design, be mixed up inextricably with the variation within treatment groups.

We would use a randomised block design which specifically recognises *both* treatment variation *and* age group (i.e. block) variation.

The results are analysed by 'analysis of variance' as before. This time the total variance displayed across all treatments and all blocks is broken up into its components—that specifically between treatments, that specifically between blocks, and the residual. We can then tell whether significant differences are present between the treatments and between the blocks. The method thus separates out the effect due to treatment from the effect due to age ('block'). The mathematics is more complicated when presented algebraically, but is routine for statisticians and available widely in pre-written computer programs.

More complex experimental designs are possible if necessary when many factors are to be incorporated into an experiment. If possible simple trials with as little variation of relevant and background factors and as much variation of the trial treatment as possible are easier to analyse. Sometimes, however, it is more economic to carry out a trial where a range of factors are involved, each taking many levels. The more complex designs allowing several factors to vary are known as factorial experiments.

Sequential Analysis

Many trials are conducted on a pre-determined number of subjects. Sometimes, however, it is preferable not to specify in advance the sample size, but to analyse the results of a trial as they become available in sequence, looking to see if significant results are showing up. Sequential analysis is the name given to this type of trial with an ongoing assessment, and it is used for comparing two treatments given to matched pairs of patients.

Patients are considered in matched pairs. One of the pair receives the orthodox treatment A, the other a new treatment B. It is essential to have clear medical criteria for deciding whether 'success' or 'failure' has been achieved for a patient and once such criteria are established, then for any matched pair of patients the outcomes can be either success for both treatments, failure for both treatments, or success for one treatment with failure for the other. When the outcomes are equal—success or failure—the result is described as a 'tied pair' and eliminated from the analysis.

A treatment 'wins' when it is successful with one member of the pair whilst the other treatment fails. For the untied pairs, every time A 'wins' it gets a score of +1, and every time B 'wins' it receives −1. For example, after seven untied pairs in which A has had six successes and B has had one success, the total 'score' would be 5, representing the advantage to A. When the number of 'advantage A' points exceeds a certain pre-set level, then we conclude that such an advantage is extremely unlikely to have occurred purely by chance, and hence A is a better treatment. The trial is then stopped. The scores are usually plotted on a graph with a boundary line beyond which A is deemed to have a significant advantage, another boundary line beyond which B has significant advantage, and a region in which we conclude that there is no difference between the treatments. The trial may be stopped as soon as a boundary line is reached, because this indicates a high advantage has built up by one of the treatments, or there is no difference between the treatments.

It should be clear that delay in evaluating new treatments is kept down, because *without* fixed size samples we do not need to wait for sufficient patients to be available to fill what is essentially an arbitrary quota in a fixed size sample. The trial using sequential analysis can be stopped as soon as a 'result' is available, and because the 'advantage' score is plotted simply onto a graph, there is no calculation for the researchers to do. The design of the experiment and the drawing of the boundary lines, however, need to be carried out by a statistician.

Sequential analysis is particularly useful where a result in favour of a new treatment is urgently sought because the existing methods have a poor prognosis. In such a case the ethics of the situation demand that the 'inferior' treatment be discontinued as soon as possible. However, it should be remembered that the data coming from a sequential trial is highly simplified, to be a cumulative preference without the full range of reported physiological measurements, comparisons and consideration of side effects.

8

Correlation and Regression Analysis

Introduction

With the advent of small computers and powerful electronic calculators, the techniques of regression and correlation analysis are in increasing use. Complicated calculation procedures can be bypassed simply by pressing a key. Correlation analysis is particularly useful in measuring the extent to which two or more variables show associated movements, and regression analysis is the method whereby the links between the variables are estimated. Regression methods also underlie a number of useful trend projection techniques.

Correlation methods are usually used where 'cause–effect' situations are under study. Cause and effect between the variables which are believed to be related needs to be established if possible prior to statistical analysis, which in itself can only assess 'association'. The relationship between cigarette smoking and lung cancer is a well-known and contentious example. Cigarette consumption might be the 'explanatory' variable, and incidence of cancer the 'dependent' variable. The causality is feasible, but the possibility of underlying factors creating both the need to smoke and the conditions for the development of cancer make straightforward application of correlation and regression analysis hazardous, when cause–effect inferences are sought.

Conditions for Use of Correlation and Regression

Ideally, simple linear regression and correlation should be used in experimental situations where the 'explanatory' variable is under the direct control of the researcher, and the effects of changes in this variable on the 'dependent' variable are measurable without error. All other factors which could affect the dependent variable should be held constant during the experiment. If data are only available historically without full control over other possible 'explanatory' variables, then multiple regression and correlation methods can incorporate extra 'explanatory' variables, provided measures on them have been recorded.

Spurious Correlation

We commence our discussion with an example of spurious correlation based on data published on death rates and smoking. The data in Table 23 relate to the number of cigarettes per adult smoked in 1930, and the standardised death rate per million per year in 1952 for 16 countries. The graph is plotted in Fig. 19, with cigarette consumption along the horizontal (the 'x' axis) and death rates

Table 23

Some International Statistics on Smoking and Death Rates

	Cigarettes Smoked Per Adult Per Annum in 1930	Death Rate in 1952
England and Wales	1 378	461
Finland	1 662	433
Austria	960	380
Netherlands	632	276
Belgium	1 066	254
Switzerland	706	236
New Zealand	478	216
USA	1 296	202
Denmark	465	179
Australia	504	177
Canada	760	176
France	585	140
Italy	455	110
Sweden	388	89
Norway	359	77
Japan	723	40

Reproduced with permission from: Doll R., Hill A.B., Gray P.G., Parr E.A. (1959). Lung cancer mortality and the length of cigarette ends. *Brit. Med. J*; February.

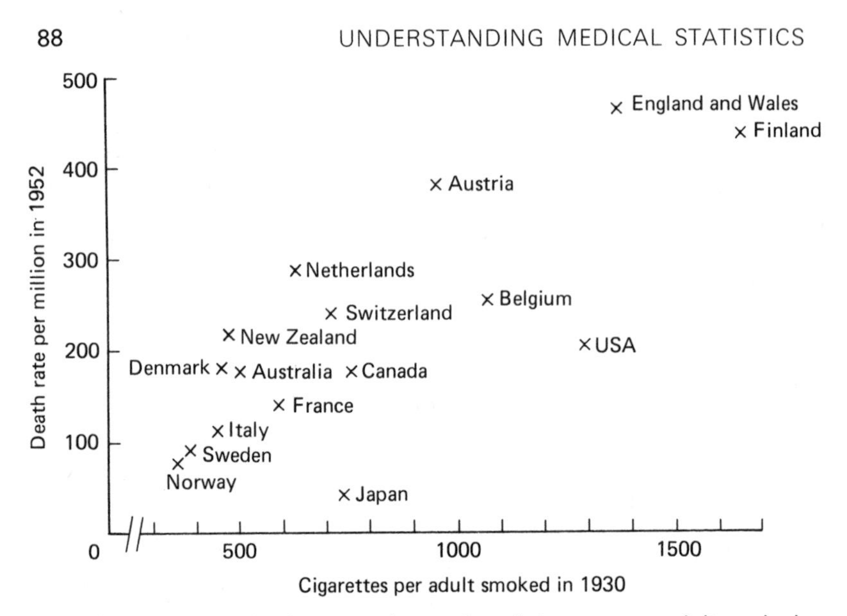

Fig. 19. The relationship between the number of cigarettes per adult smoked in 1930 and the death rate per million per year in 1952.

along the vertical (the '*y*' axis). This graph is referred to as a scatter diagram.

There appears to be a fairly clear upward-sloping relationship between smoking and cancer incidence. It is possible to take a ruler and fit a straight line by eye, and hence subjectively, to the data points on the graph, passing through as many points as possible, and minimising the distances from others. The techniques of 'simple linear regression analysis' provide an objective best-fitting line to such a set of data points, keeping the errors of the points around the line to a minimum. Correlation, or more precisely, the 'coefficient of simple correlation' is a measure of how well the points fit the line; a high correlation indicating a good fit.

The correct 'regression' line is illustrated in Fig. 20 and at face value would suggest a clear relation such that, in general, in countries with high smoking levels, greater death rates result. Further analysis of the data, however, brings out sufficient doubt to ignore both the visual evidence of a reasonably well-fitting line, and the mathematical evidence which shows some considerable association between the sets of numbers. The doubts begin when we ask 'to whom do the death rates apply?'; 'are they specific to people alive and smoking in 1930?'. This is clearly not so. In fact

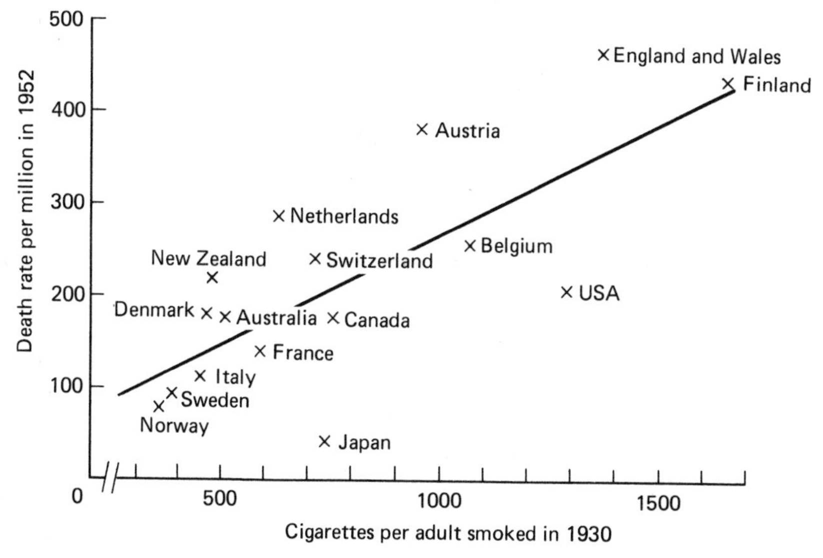

Fig. 20. The relationship between the number of cigarettes per adult smoked in 1930 and the death rate per million per year in 1952.

many people alive in 1930 would have died in that and subsequent years, for many reasons unrelated to cancer. This would be particularly true of years of war. When we turn to 1952, the deaths related to everyone who died in that year, including babies, and the many people who were not alive in 1930. The deaths are from all causes; not just cancer. The two sets of data illustrated in Fig. 19 are probably totally unrelated, and their apparent association shown graphically may be accidental, or may be caused by other factors whose nature is unspecified. What should be clear is that apparent association does not mean that proof of causality is established. Rigorous checks and questions on data definition, coverage and controls, to be fairly confident that other factors are not intervening, need to be made before inferences on causality can be legitimately sought. There needs to be sound, logical or theoretical reasons set up before a correlation analysis is made.

The Correlation Coefficient

The measure known as correlation or the 'coefficient of simple linear correlation' is numerically between 0 and 1, to indicate how well the points fit on the line. A numerical value of 1 indicates a perfect fit of points on the line, and correlation of 0 would be generated by a random scatter of points. Points on a curve can also give a simple *linear* correlation of zero, so the absence of a linear relation does not mean there is no relation. Inspection of the scatter diagram will indicate whether a curve is a better fit.

The regression line may be upward-sloping for which a correlation will be between 0 and +1, or downward-sloping for which a correlation will be between 0 and −1. A horizontal regression line may be taken as evidence of no observable relation between the variables, and a correlation of 0 would be obtained. The examples in Fig. 21 indicate some common possibilities which exist.

As a rule of thumb, a correlation of 0·6 or more yields a reasonable relationship between the variables, with the proviso that a minimum of about 12 points and preferably about 15 points is required before this is immediately acceptable. With a smaller number of points, high correlations are easily obtained by chance.

The Make-up of a Line on a Graph

Suppose we are concerned with funding a department whose daily

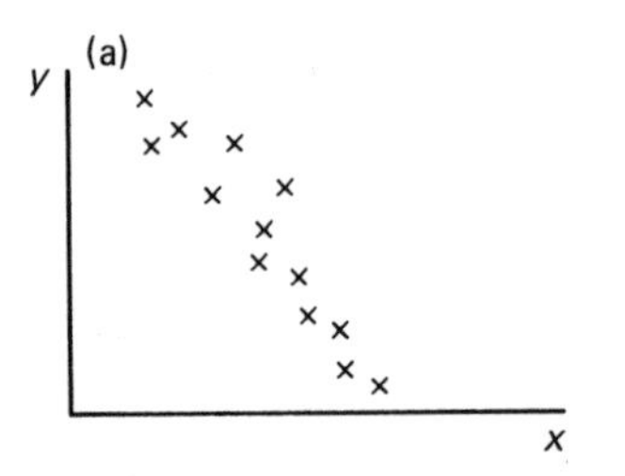

High negative correlation, close to −1

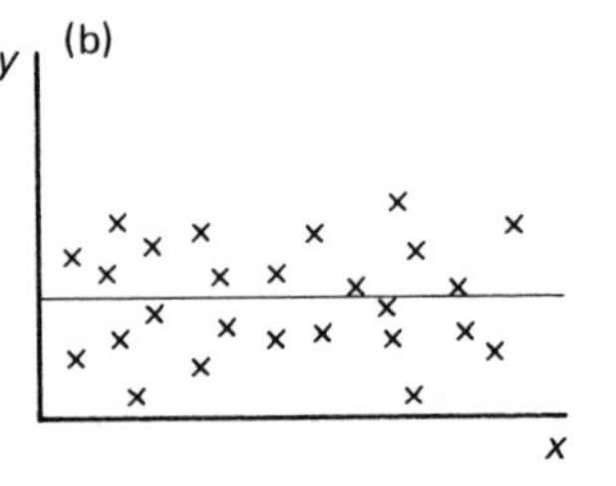

Zero correlation. The regression line is horizontal being the average value of y. There is no relation between y and x

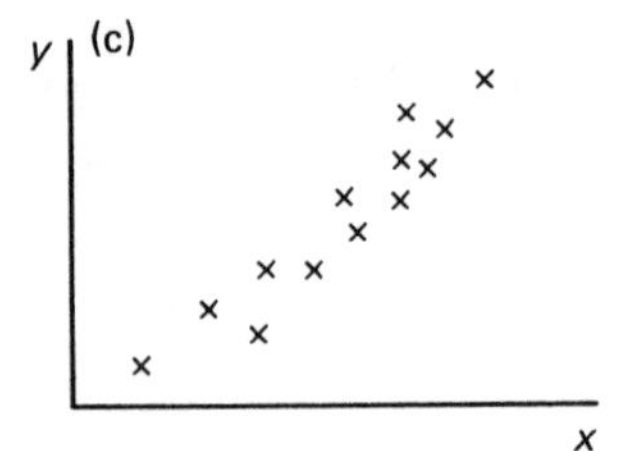

High positive correlation, close to +1

Fig. 21. Examples of positive, zero and negative correlation.

operating costs are as follows. The 'fixed' cost of opening the doors of the building (heating, lighting and basic staffing) amounts to £300 per day. Second, each patient treated is known to cost on average an extra £9, in terms of doctor's time, diagnostic procedures and treatments. Thus, if one patient only is seen per day, costs are as follows:

$$\text{Cost} = £300 + (£9 \times 1) = 309$$

If two patients are seen per day, then we have:

$$\text{Cost} = £300 + (£9 \times 2) = £318$$

If X patients are seen per day, then we have:

$$\text{Cost} = £300 + (£9 \times X)$$

Omitting the multiplication sign we have the equation for costs as:

$$\text{Cost} = 300 + 9X \quad \text{(also leaving out the £ sign)}$$

We are now in a position to use this equation to work out costs for any throughput of patients. We already have that for $X = 0$ (i.e. no patients per day), cost = £300; for $X = 1$ (i.e. 1 patient per day), cost = £309; for $X = 2$, cost = £318. In Table 24 we list the various costs for 1 to 15 patients per day, using our equation ($C = 300 + 9X$, where C is cost) to compute the values. Inspection of this table underlines the clear increase of £9 in costs for every extra patient.

Table 24

The Relationship Between Cost and Number of Patients Treated

X Number of Patients Treated	*C* Costs	*X* Number of Patients Treated	*C* Costs
0	300	8	372
1	309	9	381
2	318	10	390
3	327	11	399
4	336	12	408
5	345	13	417
6	354	14	426
7	363	15	435

We now plot a graph of cost against number of patients. Cost is the dependent variable, and is plotted on the vertical scale, and number of patients, X, is the independent variable (or explanatory variable) and is plotted on the horizontal scale. Figure 22 shows this graph to be a straight line, with the following two features:

(1) The starting point on the vertical, cost, axis is £300. This height is referred to as the 'intercept' on this axis.
(2) The line progresses upwards by £9 for every extra patient measured on the horizontal scale. This ratio (9:1) is referred to as the 'slope' (or gradient).

Whatever the position of our line, it is fully located when we know the intercept on the vertical axis for a horizontal value of zero (i.e. no patients in our example) and the slope (i.e. the extra cost per patient in our example).

If we now imagine the situation in this department where the accountants have not provided us with the information that it costs £300, merely, so to speak, to open the doors, and £9 per case; but simply, for various numbers of patients passing through, the total costs associated with this thoughput. We should probably first plot the scatter diagram, which may appear as in Fig. 23. From

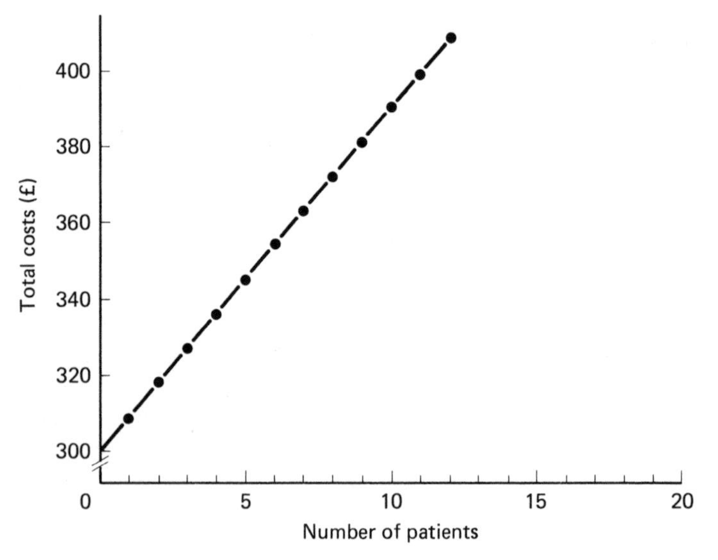

Fig. 22. Daily total costs of running a department.

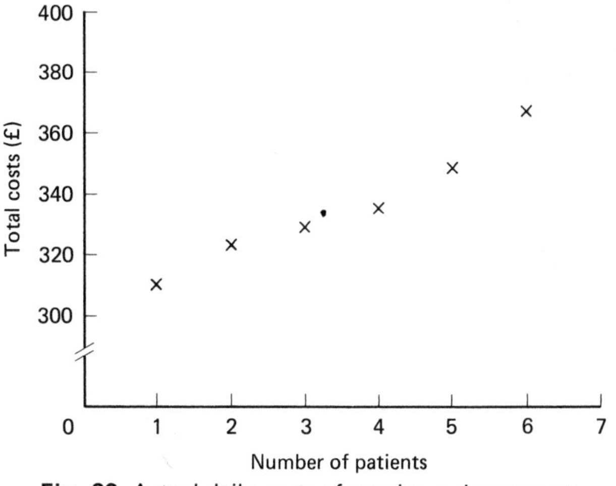

Fig. 23. Actual daily costs of running a department.

the scatter diagram we should attempt to fit a straight line to the points, which will give us the average relationship between cost and numbers. The object of a regression analysis is to locate the line, and we should seek the intercept, which of course should be around 300, and the slope, approximately 9. The exact figures 300 and 9 would be unlikely to appear because we should only have a sample of observations from which to estimate the slope and intercept, and the inherent randomness of this sort of data would be very unlikely to result, in a sample, in perfect conformity to any true underlying figures (termed 'parameters') such as 300, and 9. It is virtually certain that sampling error in each of our two estimated parameters would generate values other than 300 and 9, and when major decisions are to be made on the basis of regression results we need to have estimates of this sampling error.

Just as discussed in Chapter 5, the standard error (standard deviation) of a sample mean, and of a sample proportion, so we can calculate the standard error of a slope or an intercept. To give us some idea of the precision of our estimate we would need to be satisfied that the standard error is in fact quite low. Suppose the slope estimated from a sample of points is 8. Using our previous guidelines about the maximum error from sampling being about twice the standard error, if the latter in our example were equal to 1·5 for the slope, then our result of 8 would represent a possible true value with upper limit $8+(2\times 1{\cdot}5)=11$ and lower limit

$8-(2\times 1{\cdot}5)=5$. This would mean that the true extra cost per patient, given the data in our scatter graph, could be anything from £5 to £11 per head, although it is still true that in our sample it has averaged £8. The calculation of this standard error requires considerable work, but usually is available on computer regression programs. It should be intuitively obvious that the slope, for example, should be considerably numerically larger than its associated standard error to be in any sense precisely and reliably determined. We usually require, as a rule of thumb, that it exceed double the standard error to be statistically significant, i.e. acceptable as unlikely to have occurred purely by chance. Later in this chapter a guide to calculation for slope, intercept, correlation and standard error of the slope for situations when a computer program is not available is presented. The slope, intercept and correlation coefficient can, however, be obtained by use of some inexpensive calculators, such as the Texas Instruments T.I. 55 series, at the press of the appropriately labelled button.

Chance and Correlation

Correlation will normally be inferred from points on a scatter graph when those points appear to be along or around a line. Chance can clearly play a part in where data points fall, because we usually study a sample of possible points and so need a test to decide whether a measured and observed correlation could easily have occurred by chance. If this turns out to be the case then the correlation coefficient needs to be used with extreme caution and reservation.

If we had only two points on our scatter graph, then the line of regression would automatically pass through both and produce a perfect correlation of numerical value 1. This would hardly be acceptable, and indeed a two-point regression/correlation analysis should never be carried out! If we had three points it would, purely by chance, be quite easy for them to fall around and near to a line. For four points, again it could easily happen by chance that linear relation seems present, but as we increase to five, six, seven points, and so on, it will be more difficult for chance to distribute the points along a line.

By the time we were dealing with, say, 30 points, it would be extremely unlikely that pure chance could throw up a scatter along and close to a line.

Putting this another way, we should not read too much into a high correlation derived from a small number of points, but as the number of points increases we can be more convinced that there is real correlation present, with chance playing less of a role. In Appendix 3e the table of correlation coefficients gives the approximate highest numerical values of a correlation coefficient that could be observed generated purely by chance. The column labelled '10% significance level' means that there is a 10% probability that pure chance could provide a numerical correlation which attains or exceeds the value in the table. The columns for 1% and 5% significance levels mean that there is a 1% or 5% probability, respectively, that pure chance could provide a numerical correlation which attains or exceeds the tabulated value. Obviously, all three columns could be regarded as 'test' levels and we could compare our computed correlation coefficients in any example to assess whether they exceed the 'chance' values. If they do, we regard them as 'statistically significant' at either the 10% level, the 5% level, or the 1% level, according to which tabulated value is exceeded. Obviously, the 1% level represents a more significant result.

Inspection of Appendix 3e will reveal that for small numbers of points on the scatter graph, a very high correlation can easily be observed, and should be exceeded for us to confidently accept the correlation. Thus, for four points, at the 1% level, it is possible to observe by chance a correlation as high as 0·990. If, on the other hand, we had 17 points, then the highest chance value would be 0·482. (Strictly speaking there is actually a 1% probability of numerically exceeding 0·990 and 0·482, respectively, purely by chance.)

The fact that a correlation coefficient may be less than the tabulated value does not mean that it should be automatically discounted. The fact that it could have occurred by chance does not actually mean it did occur by chance. There exists the possibility that it is a true correlation, and hence may be judged to be indicative of a relationship, with due caution because of the lack of statistical significance.

The reader may reasonably ask why we do not always use 1% as this is the most stringent requirement. The answer lies in the high chance in this case of actually dismissing as insignificant a true correlation which may be present but less than the 1% tabulated value. The more stringent demand we made that correlations exceed possible chance values, the more likely it is that genuine correlations which are a little below these values will be rejected. The choice of the 5% significance level is most common because this represents a compromise between the extreme stringency of the 1% level and the lesser requirement of the 10% level.

It was suggested earlier in this chapter that a rule of thumb for judging the significance of a correlation coefficient was that if a minimum of 12 points were used, and a correlation of at least 0·6 showed up, then chance was unlikely to have generated the correlation. Consulting Appendix 3e we see that the exact counterpart to this rule of thumb is that for 12 points, the correlation should exceed 0·576, and for 15 points 0·514. For 'large' samples, i.e. a scatter of 30 or more points, correlations to be exceeded are not individually tabulated, but may be obtained approximately as follows. If we had a sample of 53 points, and were using the 5% significance level, we could obtain the critical values for 50 points and 60 points from Appendix 3e and estimate where 53 should come. For 50 points the test value is 0·235 and for 60 points it is 0·215. As we want 53, this is 3/10 of the distance from 50 to 60 and so we go 3/10 of the way from 0·235 to 0·215, which is 3/10 of 0·020 which is 0·006. The uppermost answer is then 0·235 – 0·006 = 0·229. This process is known as 'interpolation'.

We have continually referred to the 'numerical' value of correlation. This in effect ignores whether we have negative (inverse) correlation or positive correlation. For the purpose of checking 'statistical significance' we ignore the minus sign of negative correlation as the concept of significance applies to both, and it would be uneconomic to duplicate table entries of the identical but negative values.

Appendix 3e shows test values when we seek correlation without being specific in our thoughts in advance as to whether the correlation is negative (inverse) or positive. If we are testing, because of prior reasoning, for a positive correlation (as opposed to any kind of correlation) then it is possible to divide the significance levels by 2.

Putting this another way, figures from the 10% column become significant at 5% , figures from 5% become significant at 2·5%, and figures from the 1% column become 0·5% significance levels. The whole procedure thus becomes stronger as the significance levels decrease. Testing for specific positive (or specific negative) correlation, as distinct from correlation in general is referred to as 'one-tailed' testing, and requires considerable prior conviction about the nature of the correlation. A final cautionary note: to use the test values of correlation in Appendix 3e, we need the assumption of normally distributed data.

Examples of Simple Regression and Correlation

The examples in this section will illustrate the appearance of different levels of correlation and demonstrate some practical uses of the regression line.

An example of inverse correlation

The first example, shown in Fig. 24, is the relationship between the incomes of dentists aged over 40, and their age, taken from data from the report of the Royal Commission on Doctors' and Dentists' renumeration (1960). The data in Table 25 are in age groups, and for the purpose of analysis dentists aged 40 to 44 are assumed to be on average 42·5 years old, those aged 45 to 49 are assumed to be on average 47·5 years old, and so on. Since income depends very probably on age (and certainly not age on income) we regard income as the 'dependent' variable, to be plotted on the vertical scale, and age as the 'independent' variable on the horizontal scale. The points are seen to lie almost perfectly on the regression line, and the correlation is 'inverse' (negative), and almost perfect (−0·99). It is of course good practice to have more than five data points, but sometimes data availability is limited, as in this example. To check that this sort of correlation is unlikely to occur by chance, it should be compared with the values shown in Appendix 3e. As long as the value −0·99 numerically exceeds the relevant tabulated value (here 0·878) then it is safe to assume the correlation is 'significant' (i.e. is very unlikely to occur purely by chance).

Having obtained the line, extrapolation is carried out to produce the dotted section in Fig. 24. Here common sense must be carefully applied. It would not, for example, be sensible to project the line to work out the likely income of a dentist aged 102·5! The line suggests a negative income which implies that the dentist pays his client, rather than the usual client paying dentist. This

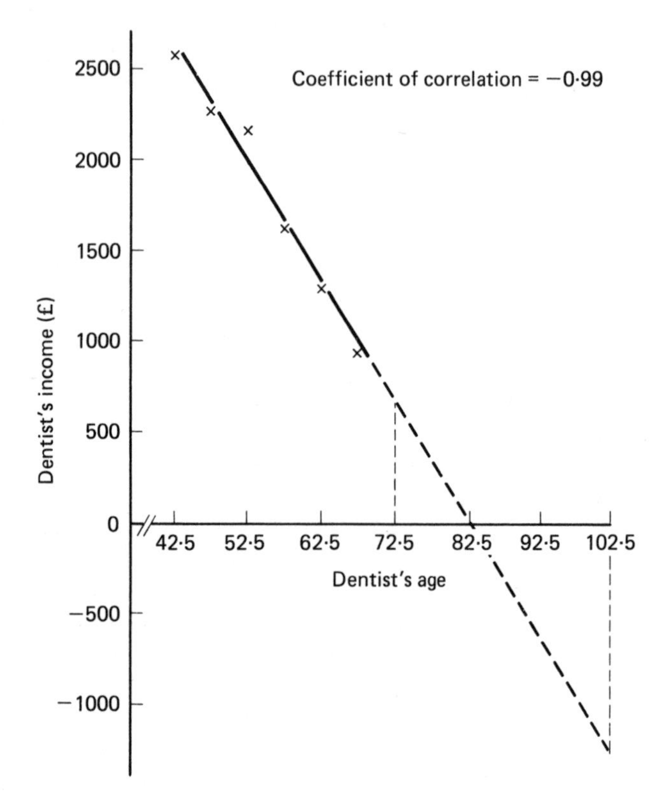

Fig. 24. The relationship between a dentist's age and his income for dentists aged over 40.

Table 25

Income of Dentists, 1955–59

Age	40–44	45–49	50–54	55–59	60–64	65–69
Average income	2 570	2 260	2 150	1 620	1 330	940

Data taken from Report of the Royal Commission on Doctors' and Dentists' Renumeration (Cmmd. 939,1960).

may be true, but 102·5 is far beyond the range of experience of ages that such a projection is unsafe. On the other hand, it is not unreasonable to project up to the age of 72·5 by reading off the income level where the projected line meets the ordinate erected at 72·5. As in all regression work, some extrapolation is reasonable, but care is required and the commonsense rejection of long extrapolations is left to the doctor's own discretion. One famous study concerned with the emptying of Britain's large psychiatric hospitals carried out a long extrapolation of the downward trend of inpatient numbers, up to the point where none would be left and the hospitals empty, and the result was duly published. This kind of obvious error—presupposing the indefinite continuation of a trend—brings statistics into undeserved disrepute.

The data in Table 26 show a man's weight loss during 21 weeks on a diet in hospital. There is an obvious downward trend (shown by Fig. 25) and the coefficient of simple linear correlation between weight and time, which is measured in weeks starting at 0, is −0·985. The intercept at week 0 is 204·08 lb, and the slope is −0·870, which indicates that the mean weekly loss in weight is 0·87 lb. Projecting the line of regression for a few weeks will probably be acceptable, and indeed could be used to check whether the weight loss was keeping to the known pattern. For example, the projection at week 30 is 177·98. Going to extremes, the formula

Table 26

Weekly Weight Loss for a Patient on a Special Diet

Week	Weight (lb)	Week	Weight (lb)
0	204	11	193
1	202	12	193
2	203	13	193
3	201	14	191
4	200	15	192
5	202	16	191
6	200	17	190
7	199	18	188
8	196	19	188
9	196	20	186
10	195		

Adapted, with permission, from *Nursing Times*, April 18, 1979.

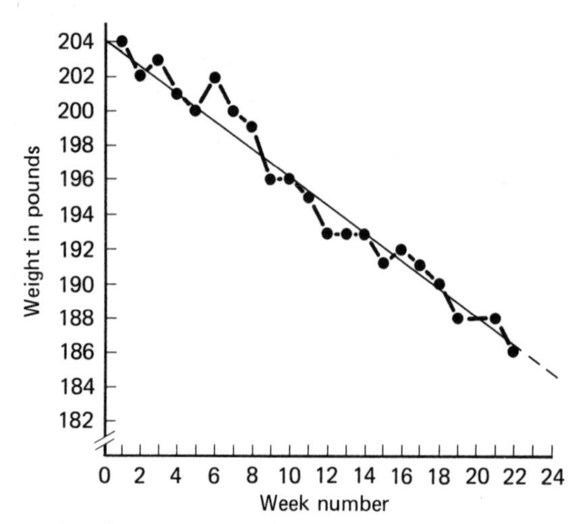

Fig. 25. Regression line used as a trend for weekly weight loss for a patient on a diet.

Table 27
Income and Diastolic Blood Pressure for 24 Male Subjects Age 40–45 (Fictitious Data)

Subject	Income (nearest 100)	Diastolic Pressure
A	3 800	60
B	4 000	65
C	4 900	63
D	5 700	75
E	6 500	66
F	7 100	73
G	7 500	72
H	7 700	75
I	8 000	72
J	8 000	74
K	8 100	76
L	8 200	64
M	8 200	73
N	8 700	75
O	9 300	80
P	9 900	77
Q	10 300	78
R	11 600	92
S	12 300	84
T	13 000	90
U	13 800	91
V	15 200	97
W	16 100	100
X	17 300	100

Coefficient of simple correlation = 0·949.

predicts that the man will disappear (have zero weight) in about 235 weeks from the start of his diet. Somewhere in between the end of week 20 and week 235, judgement must be interposed to ignore subsequent projections.

Table 27 shows the income and the diastolic blood pressure for 24 male subjects aged 40 to 45. The pronounced upward slope of the graph in Fig. 26, and the close proximity of the points to the line are noteworthy. This proximity is reflected in the high positive correlation of 0·949 which is obtained.

Calculation of slope, intercept and simple correlation

In the problem of regression we do not know the magnitude of the slope or the intercept. Thus, the problem becomes to find the values of the slope and the intercept, such that the line obtained is the best-fitting one. The formulae derived by calculus methods for slope and intercept are as follows:

$$\text{Slope} = \frac{\begin{pmatrix}\text{Number of}\\ \text{points}\end{pmatrix} \times \begin{pmatrix}\text{Sum of each } x\\ \text{multiplied by}\\ \text{its paired } y\end{pmatrix} - \begin{pmatrix}\text{Sum of}\\ \text{all } x\end{pmatrix} \times \begin{pmatrix}\text{Sum of}\\ \text{all } y\end{pmatrix}}{\begin{matrix}(\text{Number of}\\ \text{points})\end{matrix} \times \begin{matrix}\text{Sum of the squares}\\ \text{of each } x\end{matrix} - \begin{matrix}\text{Square of sum}\\ \text{of the } x\end{matrix}}$$

$$\text{Intercept} = \left(\frac{\text{Sum of all } y}{\text{Number of points}}\right) - \begin{pmatrix}\text{Slope as found}\\ \text{above}\end{pmatrix} \times \left(\frac{\text{Sum of all } x}{\text{Number of points}}\right)$$

The formula for r, the coefficient of simple correlation is:

$$r = \text{Slope} \times \frac{\begin{matrix}\text{Square}\\ \text{root of}\end{matrix} \left\{ \begin{pmatrix}\text{Number}\\ \text{of}\\ \text{points}\end{pmatrix} \times \begin{pmatrix}\text{Sum of squares}\\ \text{of each } x\\ \text{value}\end{pmatrix} - \begin{pmatrix}\text{Square of the}\\ \text{sum of all } x\\ \text{values}\end{pmatrix} \right\}}{\begin{matrix}\text{Square}\\ \text{root of}\end{matrix} \left\{ \begin{pmatrix}\text{Number}\\ \text{of}\\ \text{points}\end{pmatrix} \times \begin{pmatrix}\text{Sum of squares}\\ \text{of each } y\\ \text{value}\end{pmatrix} - \begin{pmatrix}\text{Square of the}\\ \text{sum of all } y\\ \text{values}\end{pmatrix} \right\}}$$

Since modern calculators provide intercept, slope and correlation automatically, the use of formulae can frequently be avoided.

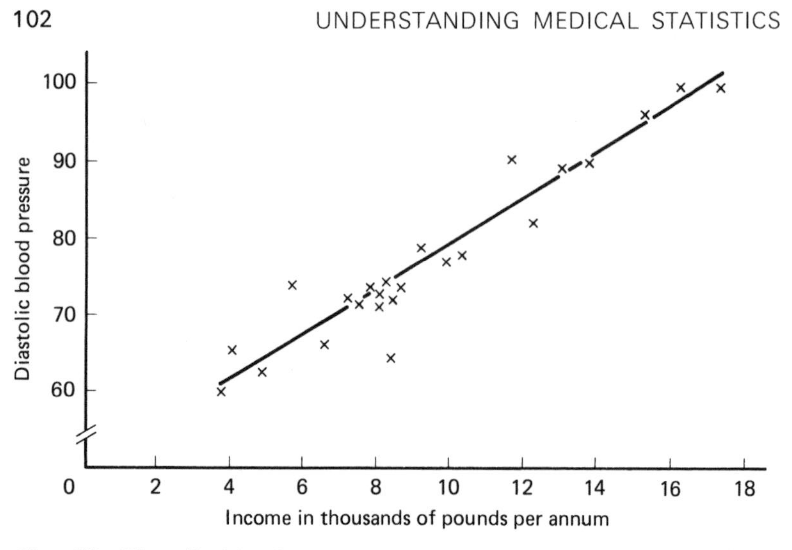

Fig. 26. Diastolic blood pressure against income (males aged 40–44, fictitious data).

The details required for obtaining the formulae for slope and intercept need not concern us, but the general principle underlying the choice of slope and intercept should be known. The line we choose should be, intuitively, one which minimises the distances between the points on the scatter graph and the line. These vertical distances (shown in Fig. 27) are referred to as 'errors', and based on these we clearly need a measure or an index of total error.

Vertical distances from points to line (labelled e_1, e_2, e_3, etc. in Fig. 27) are both positive and negative and thus the algebraic sum of errors would cancel out to zero and not give a measure of total error. Instead the errors are squared and then added, a familiar statistical device. This total sum of squares is an index of the fit of the line. A line fitted through the points which has small errors would yield a small sum of squares of these errors. Conversely, a line which fitted badly would yield numerically large errors and hence a large value of the sum of their squares. Thus, if an alternative line can be fitted with a smaller sum of squares of error this is to be preferred. It is not necessary to use trial and error methods to locate the 'best' line in this sense. Simple calculus methods yield the formula shown above for the equations of the

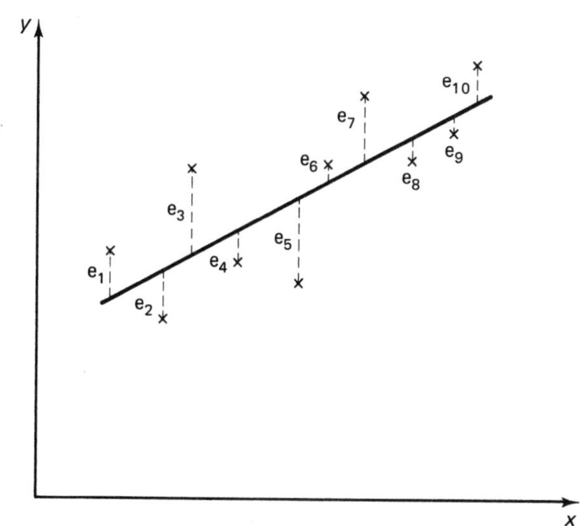

Fig. 27. The 'errors' around a regression line.

Table 28

Data for Regression and Correlation Calculation

x	y	x	y	x	y
1	3	4	14	7	26
2	5	5	17	8	29
3	9	6	19	9	35

slope and intercept of the line with the least sum of squares of error, and hence best fit. The regression line is thus frequently referred to as the 'least squares' line.

Whilst the use of either a computer regression program, or a calculator such as the Texas Instruments T.I. 55 Series, is strongly recommended, it is nevertheless sometimes necessary to calculate a slope, intercept and correlation coefficient using the formulae. Accordingly, a layout of the calculation for the following data is offered. x is the independent variable, and y is the dependent variable, and a clear upward-sloping relation is suggested by inspecting the data of Table 28. The formula indicates that we require the following quantities:

(1) Number of 'points', i.e. pairs of x, y values. This is nine in the example.

(2) Sum of each x multiplied by its paired y. The calculation becomes:

x	y	(x times y)
1	3	3
2	5	10
3	9	27
4	14	56
5	17	85
6	19	114
7	26	182
8	29	232
9	35	315

Sum of (x times y) = 1 024

(3) Sum of all $x = 45$
Sum of all $y = 157$

(4) The sum of the squares of each x value is calculated thus:

x	Squares of x
1	1
2	4
3	9
4	16
5	25
6	36
7	49
8	64
9	81

Sum of squares of x values = 285

The sum of the squares of each y value is calculated thus:

y	Squares of y
3	9
5	25
9	81
14	196
17	289
19	361
26	676
29	841
35	1 225

Sum of squares of y values = 3 703

(5)

$$\text{Slope} = \frac{(9 \times 1024) - (45 \times 157)}{(9 \times 285) - (45 \times 45)}$$

$$= \frac{9216 - 7065}{2565 - 2025}$$

$$= \frac{2151}{540}$$

$$= 3{\cdot}9833$$

(6)

$$\text{Intercept} = \frac{157}{9} - 3{\cdot}9833 \times \frac{45}{9}$$

$$= 17{\cdot}4444 - 19{\cdot}9165$$

$$= -2{\cdot}4721$$

(7)

$$\text{Correlation} = \frac{3{\cdot}9833 \times \text{Square root of } ((9 \times 285) - (45 \times 45))}{\text{Square root of } ((9 \times 3703) - (157 \times 157))}$$

$$= \frac{3{\cdot}9833 \times \text{Square root of } 540}{\text{Square root of } 8678}$$

$$= \frac{3{\cdot}9833 \times 23{\cdot}2379}{93{\cdot}1558}$$

$$= \frac{92{\cdot}5635}{93{\cdot}1558}$$

$$= 0{\cdot}9936$$

The results of the calculation give the equation of the regression line as:

$$y = -2{\cdot}4721 + 3{\cdot}9833x$$

From this equation we can draw the line through the scatter of points on our graph by working out any y value corresponding to any chosen x value. For example, when $x = 1$, then:

$$\begin{aligned} y &= -2{\cdot}4721 + (3{\cdot}9833 \times 1) \\ &= 1{\cdot}5112 \end{aligned}$$

When $x = 2$, then:

$$\begin{aligned} y &= -2{\cdot}4721 + (3{\cdot}9833 \times 2) \\ &= 5{\cdot}4945 \end{aligned}$$

and so on. Table 29 lists all the 'predicted' y values, which are the vertical distances from the x axis to our line, and also lists the actual y values so that we may compare and assess the errors.

Correlation 'explained'

At this point it is interesting to pause and reflect on what our correlation and regression analysis is doing. We have a variable x which takes values from one to nine, and is believed to cause another variable y to vary, in this case from 3 to 35. It is our object then to explain this variability in y and account for it by the movements of x and the use of connecting 'link' $y = -2{\cdot}4721 + 3{\cdot}9833x$. Having established this 'link', it produces the 'predicted' values shown in Table 29.

Table 29

Comparison of 'Actual' y Value with 'Predicted' y Value from the Regression Equation

x	y Predicted	y Actual
1	1·511 2	3
2	5·494 5	5
3	9·477 8	9
4	13·461 1	14
5	17·444 4	17
6	21·427 8	19
7	25·411 1	26
8	29·394 4	29
9	33·377 8	35

Clearly it should be our expectation that the variation shown in the actual y values is very closely mirrored by the variation obtained in the 'predicted' y values. If exactly identical variation were obtained, then this would be highly satisfactory and give considerable confidence to the user of the regression equation. It would mean that we are matching the variation in the observed y by our prediction, and we are in a sense 'explaining' the variation in y in terms of x and the linking formula.

We can actually measure the variation in y by calculating its variance, or its standard deviation. The variance of y works out to be 107·1358, and its standard deviation, as the square root of this, is 10·350. Now if we compute the variance and standard deviation for the 'predicted' y values we should hopefully obtain very similar values. The variance of the predicted y values is 105·7791, and the standard deviation 10·2849. Comparing first the variances: for the predictions it is 105·7791 and for the actual values 107·1358. Thus, for the amount of variation to be 'explained', 107·1358, we have successfully accounted for 105·7791, or as a proportion, $105{\cdot}7791/107{\cdot}1358 = 0{\cdot}9873$. This value is known as the coefficient of determination, which is now interpreted as the proportion of the variance of the dependent variable which is 'explained' by the regression. The coefficient of determination is often referred to as 'r squared'. Frequently, it is converted to a percentage: we would say that $0{\cdot}9873 \times 100 = 98{\cdot}73\%$ of variance of the dependent variable is explained by the regression.

As an alternative and much less common comparison, we note that the standard deviation of the actual values of the dependent variable is 10·3506, and the standard deviation of the 'predicted' values is 10·2849. Dividing 10·2849 by 10·3506 produces the value 0·9936 which will be recognised as the level of the coefficient of simple correlation obtained more directly earlier in this chapter.

To obtain the value of the simple correlation in any practical situation the most efficient calculation procedure is to use the formula presented earlier in the section on calculation of slope, intercept and simple correlation. This has the advantage that the correct sign (plus or minus) is automatically produced. In the explanation in terms of proportion of the variance explained we went on to take a square root, which could of course be plus or minus. To know which would involve plotting the scatter diagram and deciding by looking whether the points sloped up to the right or down to the left.

Mathematically, the coefficient of determination is more attractive to handle than its square root and, can be obtained directly by squaring the coefficient of simple correlation.

The Sampling Error in a Regression Slope

When we assess the value of a regression, one of the most important factors is the extent to which we can rely on the slope to be precise and close to the true value which would be obtained if all the possible data, rather than just our sample, were used.

The standard error of the slope can be estimated, and from it we can obtain a confidence interval for the true slope. The calculation procedure is shown below, but the derivation of the formula is omitted because of its mathematical complexity. Using the data of Table 30, we need to construct three numbers, which we will call A, B, and C. Having obtained these, the variance of the slope is then estimated as $A \div B \div C$, and the standard deviation (or more precisely 'standard error') as the square root of $(A \div B \div C)$.

'A' is the sum of squares of the (vertical) deviations of errors of the scatter graph points from the regression line. 'B' is two less than the number of points in the scatter. 'C' is the sum of the squared deviations of the x values from their mean.

Table 30

Table Used in Calculation of Sampling Error in a Regression Slope

x	y	'Predictions'	Error = y-Prediction	Squares of Errors	Deviations of x from Mean	Squared Deviations of x from Mean
1	3	1·5112	1·4888	2·2165	−4	16
2	5	5·4945	−0·4945	0·2445	−3	9
3	9	9·4778	−0·4778	0·2283	−2	4
4	14	13·4611	0·5389	0·2904	−1	1
5	17	17·4444	−0·4444	0·1975	0	0
6	19	21·4278	−2·4278	5·8942	1	1
7	26	25·4111	0·5889	0·3468	2	4
8	29	29·3944	−0·3944	0·1556	3	9
9	35	33·3778	1·6222	2·6315	4	16
				A = sum = 12·2054		C = sum = 60

We have already obtained the slope as 3·9833, the intercept as −2·4721 and the coefficient of simple correlation as 0·9936. We also have the 'heights' to the line (which we call predictions), shown in Table 29 and again in Table 30. The calculation procedure for the variance or standard error of a regression coefficient now follows. We first construct a column labelled 'errors', these being each actual y value minus the predicted (line) value. We then square each error in the next column, and add the entries in this column. The sum is A. Next we note that there are nine points on the scatter graph, so B is $9-2=7$. We now construct a column showing the deviation of each x value from the mean. The mean of the x values is 5, so each entry is the appropriate x minus 5. The final column is the square of each deviation, and these are added to produce C. It can be seen that A = 12·2054, B = 7, and C = 60. Accordingly, the variance of the regression slope is 12·2054 ÷ 7 ÷ 60 = 0·029 06. Hence the standard error is the square root, which is 0·1705. Accordingly our regression coefficient (3.9833) has a standard error of 0·1705, which is relatively very small. The ratio 3·9833 ÷ 0·1705 = 23·36, indicates relatively little error, and thus that 3·9833 is well determined. If, as a rule of thumb, the ratio were less than two, then we would say that the regression slope is not significant, being of a comparable size to its standard error.

In the case of our example, the approximate 95% confidence interval for the true slope is obtained by taking the regression slope of 3·9833 and allowing an interval equal to twice the standard error around it, producing a lower possible limit of $3{\cdot}9833-(2\times0{\cdot}1705)$, and an upper limit of $3{\cdot}9833+(2\times0{\cdot}1705)$, i.e. 3·6423 to 4·3243. Further improvement can be made by altering the two to a value slightly larger, to allow for the problem of a small sample of observations. The appropriate value would be read from a t table, but care must be taken to read from the 95% column and the row for degrees of freedom equal to two less than the number of points in the scatter diagram, because by estimating both slope and intercept from the sample data we have used up two degrees of freedom. The table gives the value 2·365 to replace the two used in the confidence interval above, and thus widens it to $3{\cdot}9833-(2{\cdot}365\times0{\cdot}1705)$ to $3{\cdot}9833+(2{\cdot}365\times0{\cdot}1705)$, i.e. from 3·5801 to 4·3865. Only when there are less than 30 points should we use the t values shown in Appendix 3, and then reading from the line appropriate to the degrees of freedom equal to the number of points in the scatter, less the number of parameters estimated from the data, which in the case of simple linear regression gives the degrees of freedom as number of points in the scatter less two (because we have estimated two parameters: the slope and the intercept).

Multiple Regression

Our earlier introductory example of simple linear regression related to a hospital facility offering one type of treatment, which we shall now call treatment A. Suppose it is now policy to offer additionally a completely different patient treatment programme whose costs per patient are quite unrelated to the costs for treatment A. The costs for B, over and above our £300 fixed costs, are £17 per patient; and any costs for patients on treatment A are, of course, £9 per patient. Suppose we have four patients on treatment A and five on treatment B, then our total costs are:

$$\text{Costs} = £300 + (£9 \times 4) + (£17 \times 5)$$

If we have eight patients on treatment A and four on B, then total costs are:

$$\text{Costs} = £300 + (£9 \times 8) + (£17 \times 4)$$

and if we have X patients on treatment A and Z patients on B, then costs are given by:

$$\text{Costs} = 300 + 9X + 17Z \text{ (omitting multiplication and pound signs)}$$

Just as in our previous example we worked out a list of costs for various numbers of patients on treatment A (in Table 24) so we can now compute costs for any combination of patients having treatment A or treatment B.

To plot a scatter analogous to Fig. 23 would require three axes; one for cost, one for the number of patients on treatment A, and one for the number of patients on treatment B. A three-dimensional graph would emerge, and instead of fitting a line through points in two dimensions, as in Fig. 23, we would fit a plane surface through points in three dimensions.

Suppose in our example that our accountants have not provided the figures of fixed costs, or cost per patient on treatment A and treatment B, but that only total costs have been recorded for all patients passing through the facility, and we also know the numbers having each type of treatment. We are now *not* in a position to use our equation:

$$\text{Cost} = 300 + 9X + 17Z$$

because we do not know the 300, the 9 or the 17. We need to estimate these using multiple regression methods from our sample data.

Multiple regression 'slopes'

It has already been suggested for simple regression that we would, however well we carry out our calculations, be extremely unlikely to hit upon the correct slope or intercept values, because a sample is being used and sampling error will be present in each of our estimates. As a general rule we need to know the standard error of each of the two 'slopes' we estimate, these slopes being the additional costs per person for treatments A and B. We need to be satisfied that these standard errors are small in relation to the estimates of the slopes we obtain. The technique of multiple regression provides, analogously to simple linear regression, values of the slopes which are the best possible in the circumstances. These values, as a rule of thumb, need to be at least double the standard error estimated for each of them. The calculation of standard error is best left to a computer program, but it is an essential piece of information when we come to evaluate multiple regression results. For example, suppose the multiple regression gives:

intercept—210
slope, treatment A—5·3
slope, treatment B—18·4
standard error of slope, treatment A—0·2
standard error of slope, treatment B—0·9

The estimated equation for cost is then:

$$\text{Cost} = 210 + 5{\cdot}3X + 18{\cdot}4Z$$

However, remembering that the approximate maximum error from sampling is about twice the standard error, in the case of the value 5·3, it may represent a true value in the range

$$5{\cdot}3 - (2 \times 0{\cdot}2) \text{ to } 5{\cdot}3 + (2 \times 0{\cdot}2), \text{ i.e. } 4{\cdot}9 \text{ to } 5{\cdot}7$$

Thus, the estimated cost per extra patient using treatment A is expected to be between £4·9 and £5·7. Similarly for treatment B, the value 18·4 may very well represent a true value in the range

$$18{\cdot}4 - (2 \times 0{\cdot}9) \text{ to } 18{\cdot}4 + (2 \times 0{\cdot}9), \text{ i.e. } 16{\cdot}6 \text{ to } 20{\cdot}2$$

Thus, extra patients using treatment B cost anywhere from £16·6 to £20·2 per head. It should be clear that the standard errors of the slopes are vital pieces of information, all too often omitted in reported research. Suppose that the information from a multiple regression computer program based on analysis of a large amount of data (i.e. sufficient to satisfy us of its representativeness) gives

intercept—210
slope, treatment A—5·3
slope, treatment B—18·4
standard error, treatment A—4·7
standard error, treatment B—12·8

The simple criterion that a slope should be at least double standard error is not satisfied and if we were to work out confidence limits, as in the previous example, they would be so wide as to be useless. Thus, the regression equation could not be used with any reliability.

Multicollinearity

A factor which further reduces the reliability of regression slopes (usually called regression coefficients) is a phenomenon known as multicollinearity. Putting this briefly, it occurs when the explanatory variables, such as numbers of patients having treatments A and B, are themselves highly correlated. Sometimes, when we have more than two explanatory variables, whole clusters of them may themselves be heavily intercorrelated. This means that they all tend to move in the same direction. Supposing this to be in the same direction as the dependent variable, in our case costs, there is no reliable way we can ascribe changes in costs to unit changes in a particular explanatory variable. In short, we cannot believe the regression coefficients; they have large standard errors, and should not determine policy.

An example of the type of multiple regression work which can suffer seriously from the problems of highly intercorrelated groups or pairs of explanatory variables (i.e. multicollinearity) is work related to nurse staffing. In the midwifery field, for example, a sample of 100 units yielded the following multiple regression equation:

$$\begin{aligned}\text{Number of whole-time equivalent midwives and pupil midwives}\\ = 0{\cdot}337 + (0{\cdot}001\,27 \times \text{Number of births})\\ + (0{\cdot}660 \times \text{Number of occupied beds})\\ + (0{\cdot}000\,89 \times \text{Total outpatient attendances})\end{aligned}$$

The implications for staffing are that one more birth adds 0·00127 midwives to the required complement; that one more occupied bed adds 0·660 midwives; and that one more outpatient requires 0·000 89 midwives. If the number of births was unrelated to the number of occupied beds, which in turn was unrelated to outpatient attendances, then we might be able to use the figures 0·001 27, 0·660 and 0·000 89 to help in establishing overall staffing norms, and to indicate which units are over- or under-staffed relative to the 'predictions' that the equation gives. Unfortunately, a simple correlation analysis between births and occupied beds gives the correlation coefficient as 0·97, i.e. almost perfect; between births and outpatient attendances as 0·86; and between occupied beds and attendances as 0·89. This intercorrelation means that the number of midwives correlates well with any one, any two or all three of the explanatory variables and that no reliance can be placed on the regression coefficients, which are intended to measure the particular contribution of the variable to which they are attached.

Putting this another way, the slopes (regression coefficients) have a large amount of standard error associated with them and are unreliable. Thus, the value 0·001 27 has a standard error of 0·003 93, which is three times as large as the slope, meaning that the approximate true upper limit in the population of all such units is $0{\cdot}00127 + (2 \times 0{\cdot}00393) = 0{\cdot}00913$, and the approximate lower limit is $-0{\cdot}00659$. According to the regression analysis, the contribution of one more birth, on average within our sample, is 0·001 27 midwives, but the extension of the result to all possible midwifery units leaves us with the possibility that it is as high as 0·009 midwives, and could actually be negative at −0·006 59! It will be recalled that the range −0·006 59 to 0·009 13 is called a confidence interval, and given that the 'coefficient' for 'number of occupied beds' is 0·660 with standard error 0·1525 we obtain the range $0{\cdot}660 - (2 \times 0{\cdot}1525)$ to $0{\cdot}660 + (2 \times 0{\cdot}1525)$, i.e. 0·355 to 0·965 as the confidence interval for the addition to the number of midwives made by one extra occupied bed. Finally, the coefficient for total outpatient attendances is 0·000 89, with standard error 0·000 33, giving the confidence interval from 0·000 23 to 0·001 55 for the number of extra midwives for each extra outpatient attendance. Given these very large variations in the possible true values it is perhaps not surprising that if another sample of 100 units is considered, the values which emerge from a regression analysis carried out on annual data are:

$$\begin{aligned}\text{Number of whole-time equivalent midwives and pupil midwives}\\ = 0{\cdot}645 + (0{\cdot}002 \quad &\times \text{Number of births})\\ + (0{\cdot}7137 \quad &\times \text{Number of occupied beds})\\ + (0{\cdot}00071 &\times \text{Total outpatient attendances})\end{aligned}$$

Whilst 0·002, 0·7137 and 0·000 71 all clearly fall within the confidence intervals calculated above, they are quite different from 0·001 27, 0·660, and 0·000 89 obtained earlier. Thus, the placing of too much faith in individual coefficients should be avoided when multicollinearity shows between 'explanatory' variables. The working out of the simple correlations between pairs of explanatory variables will show whether multicollinearity is present.

Multiple Correlation and Determination

Earlier in this chapter we discussed the meaning of simple determination, seeing it as the proportion of the variance of the dependent variable that is accounted for by the simple linear regression. Exactly analogously to this, the coefficient of multiple determination is the proportion of the variance of the dependent variable in a multiple regression equation which is 'accounted for' for the equation. Multiple determination is the variance of the 'predicted' '*Y*' values divided by the variance of the actual '*Y*' values, (where *Y* is the dependent variable) and takes values in the range 0 to 1. Multiple correlation is the square root of multiple determination and is much less widely used. Most calculations that are done in the field of multiple regression are carried out using a ready-made computer program, such as SPSS described in Chapter 11. Such programs automatically print out the value of the multiple determination, calling it 'R SQUARED', but do not bother to take the square root.

The fact that we may obtain a very high coefficient of multiple determination or correlation does not mean that all aspects of our results are definitely valid. Standard errors of regression coefficient need assessing, conditions and controls obtaining on the situation need to be satisfactory with other factors held constant or known to be largely invariant, and spurious correlation needs to be avoided.

Rank Correlation

Simple linear correlation is a measure of the closeness of association between two variables. Sometimes, however, the information on the variables is not available in the usual numerical form. If we can assign rankings to the items within each of the two variables, then a rank correlation can be calculated.

Suppose we have a theory that psychiatric patients become socially 'disabled' because of long periods of institutionalisation. If we were to test this theory we might seek to create an index of disability, and discover how this is associated with the period of time spent in hospital. Setting up the controls for this kind of study would require considerable work because the only patients to be allowed in should be as similar as possible at their time of entry to the hospital in as many factors as possible, and have received broadly similar treatment and hospital experience, so that observed differences in disability could be attributed to a long period in hospital. (A more sophisticated study might require a control group, such as psychiatric patients who are treated as outpatients, but who otherwise match the sample group, for comparison purposes.) The information required may well be old, unreliable, unavailable and imprecise. For the purposes of our example suppose that we are satisfied that ten patients we have found are broadly speaking 'matched'. We now need an index of disability, and however we measure disability some subjectivity is inevitable. Suppose our index runs from 1 to 10, with the value 10 signifying the extreme of disability. By choosing the index to have the same number of points as the number of patients we are dealing with, the index is merely a ranking of the patients, and should be relatively easy to construct. This kind of data is ordinal (i.e. has significance only according to rank order) and has been met earlier in Chapter 6 where we discussed non-parametric statistics. Recall that a patient with rank 4 is not twice as disabled as a patient with rank 2, nor is the difference in disability between them necessarily the same (in any sense) as the difference between ranks 8 and 10.

Having created our disability ranking we now examine the patients' records for length of time in hospital, and discover some ink blots on vital dates, and some illegible entries. After hunting for clues in the case notes, we conclude that the 'lengths of stay' can not be stated exactly but can be put into rank order, from 1 to 10, where 10 signifies the greatest period of continuous hospitalisation. Even if all the exact original dates were available we would still use a ranking, because we want to associate disability rank with length of stay rank. We calculate the measure of association between the ranks from a formula developed by Spearman in the early 1900s for the 'coefficient of rank correlation'. As with simple linear correlation a value of 1 shows perfect association, and hypothesis tests and tables are available to check whether the measured coefficient of rank correlation could have occurred by chance given the size of the sample taken, even if there is no real association present in 'the population'. One important advantage of rank correlation over ordinary correlation even on ordinary arithmetic data is that when some extreme observations are included in an ordinary coefficient of simple linear correlation they can have a predominating and somewhat distorting effect. Visually, they would appear as outlying points on the scatter diagram, and we might judge perhaps somewhat arbitrarily that they should be excluded from the calculation of simple correlation. No such problem exists with rank correlation, because extreme observations in ranked data will never produce a large rank difference. To illustrate, if the lengths of stay of three patients were 7, 8 and 9 years, when put into rank order we get 1, 2 and 3. If on the other hand they were 7, 8 and 62 years, when put into rank order we still get 1, 2 and 3. The extreme effect of the 62 is thus easily handled and of course 62 probably has no difference in medical terms to, for example, 39 or 47. It is simply a very long period, and is best thought of by rank. The formula works by getting the differences between the ranks of disability and of length of stay for each patient, squaring them, and working with these squares.

$$\text{Rank correlation} = 1 - \frac{6 \times \text{Sum of squared differences}}{\text{Number of paired observations} \times \left[\text{Square of number of paired observations} - 1\right]}$$

If the rank for length of stay is much the same for each patient as the rank for disability, each difference will be small and so will the sum of their squares. Hence, the rank correlation as calculated from Spearman's formula will be 1 minus a small number and hence close to 1. If, on the other hand, the ranks bear no relation to each other, then differences will be large, the squares will be large, and when they are included in Spearman's formula, will give a rank correlation close to zero.

Sometimes ties occur in the ranks. These are dealt with by ascribing as the 'rank' the average of the successive ranks that would have been given had the values been different. Thus, if three observations are equal seventh, then had they been unequal they would have been seventh, eighth and ninth. The rank given to each is eighth. The calculations for the ten patients are as shown in Table 31.

A rank correlation of 0·6 suggests a reasonable positive association between social disability and length of stay. Carrying out a one-tailed test of significance at the 5% level using the table in Appendix 3d shows that the critical value to be exceeded to

Table 31

Example of Rank Correlation, Showing Positive Association Between Social Disability and Length of Stay

Patient	Column 1 Disability Rank	Column 2 Length of Stay Rank	Col. 1 – Col. 2 Difference	Square of Difference
A	1	2	−1	1
B	4	7	−3	9
C	3	1	2	4
D	5	6	−1	1
E	2	4	−2	4
F	6	8	−2	4
G	8	9	−1	1
H	10	5	5	25
I	7	3	4	16
J	9	10	−1	1
			Sum of squares =	66

$$\text{Rank correlation} = 1 - \frac{6 \times 66}{10(100-1)} = 1 - \frac{396}{990} = 0{\cdot}6$$

persuade us that our rank correlation has not occurred just by chance is 0·5515. Hence, in this case we have enough evidence to reject the hypothesis of zero rank correlation at the 5% level. Checking at the 2·5% level (i.e. 0·025), the critical value is 0·6364 and so, if we had chosen this level at first, we should not now reject the hypothesis of no association in favour of the alternative of positive association. This problem of our test value (0·6) falling between the various usual critical values is not uncommon, and leaves us in a position of having to reserve judgement about the association. There are obvious indications of association here, but the evidence is by no means conclusive.

Conclusions

The techniques of this chapter have many applications and are well within the capability of the numerate doctor, especially when the appropriate calculator is available. The possibility that correlations could be spurious or arise by chance, and the recognition that sampling error is inherent in regression slopes and intercepts and coefficients of correlation, should temper conclusions from this type of analysis. To utilise regression and correlation safely, as much control as possible needs to be kept over the data, ensuring that reliable data are used and that significant variables other than the chosen 'explanatory' variable are not having pronounced individual effects. Where one or more other variables are believed to be highly significant in explaining the variable of interest, then the multiple regression and correlation techniques are to be preferred. When data are available historically, control is not possible and hence careful thought about the likely validity of the relationships needs to precede the analysis.

As an alternative to a correlation analysis, where one or more variables 'explain' another, the trend of a measurement such as a serum creatinine level (monthly), or number of infections reported (monthly), may be investigated. Thus, a graph with, for example, number of surgical wound infections on the vertical axis, and time on the horizontal axis, may indicate a linear upward trend. The regression is then performed with time as the independent variable. Thus, for monthly observations, if the months are labelled 0, 1, 2, 3, etc., a regression line fitted through the points will highlight the trend and predictions can be made, again taking care not to extrapolate too far into the future.

Further developments of regression include the fitting of curves to data as alternatives to straight lines, especially when some upper or lower limit to the value of the dependent variable is expected or sought. A selection of curves is available on certain modern electronic calculators equipped with 'libraries' of programs. For projections of short distances into the future a simple linear regression is usually sufficient. For longer-term projection it is advisable to fit a trend curve in addition to a line to provide an alternative forecast.

A final cautionary note applies to projecting the line of regression—a process known as 'extrapolation'. Just as we need to have confidence that a relationship has some validity prior to our analysis, so careful thought must be given to an extrapolation, and it should be remembered that long extrapolations can produce nonsensical results. The regression equation represents an observed average association between two or more variables over a limited range of their joint variation, based on a sample of data.

Inferences and projections should always be limited by judgement and common sense.

Regression and correlation have frequently been misused and thus maligned. Intelligent use with careful assessment of validity of use, puts into the hands of doctors a powerful tool for assessing the strength of cause–effect relationships and for basic projection. Results from regression analysis should not be used until after a full and critical discussion has been made of the assumptions, controls and errors involved. As with other techniques, regression and correlation do not make decisions, but rather can be one of the informational inputs, taking a place alongside other quantitative and qualitative considerations.

9

Vital Statistics

Introduction

Vital statistics are numerical items of information about some of the main events in life: birth, illness, marriage, divorce, death and so on. The concern of this chapter is to establish some of the more useful measures appertaining to those vital statistics of interest to the doctor.

Consider the statement: 'There were 279 cases of rubella'. This is not very useful until we know the nature of the population to which it relates, and the time period in which the cases were observed. To allow for different population sizes, information of this sort is usually expressed in the form of a rate per 1000 people for a particular time period. A rate is an extension of the idea of a percentage value to bases other than 100. Rates may be expressed per 1000, per 100 000, per million, or other bases dependent on the particular circumstances. In general we define a rate as the frequency of a disease or characteristic, per unit size of the population or group in which it is observed.

A rate can allow for more than one 'event' per person in the population. Thus, someone who experiences two attacks of influenza in the relevant period is included twice in calculating the influenza incidence rate, i.e. the number of influenza attacks starting in a given population in the period, related to the population size. The population 'at risk' is frequently the mid-year population when the rate is expressed relating to a year.

A rate measures the number of events occurring in a defined population in a period, in relation to the size of that population. We may conveniently imagine a flow of events, with 'rate' indicating the speed of the flow.

Some so called 'rates' are in fact simple ratios. For example, the 'case fatality rate' is the number of deaths from a particular disease, divided by the number of persons who contract that disease, and then expressed as a percentage by multiplying by 100. The case fatality rate is thus a ratio, not really a rate which flows dynamically through time.

Many so called indexes are only ratios. That is, two associated factors or attributes are measured and one is divided by the other and the result expressed as a percentage. For example, the 'vital index' for a population is the number of births related to the number of deaths—the higher the index, the higher the indicated vitality of the population. More complicated indexes may take several factors into account, with appropriate weightings according to importance to arrive at a weighted sum as the 'index', or even the ratio of two weighted sums. For example, the 'retail price index' relates 'average' price now to average price in a base period. Each average is a weighted average of all the items on which a typical household may make expenditures, weighted by relative importance.

Simpler 'indexes' exist, such as the number of hospital beds per 100 000 population, or the number of nurses per bed. In these indexes, the dynamic element implied by a rate is absent. These indexes relate to what 'is', and in fact are ratios. For a particular disease if we divide the number of persons affected by the number not affected, we obtain a ratio. If we had divided the number affected in the period by the total population at risk we would have obtained a rate.

Rates have the advantage that they are easy to use for wider comparisons, for calculations and, if needed, as 'probabilities' of incidence.

We consider in the following sections some rates and ratios that are in common use.

Fertility Rates

The (crude) 'birth rate' is the number of live births occurring in a period per 1000 population. The population is usually estimated as at mid year from census data. The birth rate would be expressed for a particular year as, for example, 17 per 1000. A birth rate could appear to be low in a population which is predominantly male or predominantly above child bearing age, even though there is nothing wrong with the fertility of those 'eligible' to have children. The 'general fertility rate' may be more useful, because it is the number of live births per 1000 women of child bearing age.

Even though the general fertility rate may be agreed on as relating, for example, to females aged 15 to 49 inclusive, the actual age distribution within this range affects the obtained rate. Accordingly, we may calculate 'age specific fertility rates' as the number of live births to women of a specific age group per 1000 women in that age group in a certain period. Thus, an overall general fertility rate of 26 per thousand may contain variation from, for example, 32 per thousand for women aged 20–24 inclusive to 14 per thousand in women 35–39 inclusive.

Suppose we followed the child bearing progress of 1000 females from the age of 15, applying to them the age specific fertility rate for each age group until they reached 49. This group—known as a 'cohort'—might perhaps theoretically bear a total of 3400 children. Thus, the average number of babies born to a woman in her child bearing period is 3·4, or it may be expressed per 1000 as 3400. This figure is referred to as the 'total fertility rate'.

Following the approach of the 'total fertility rate', but referring to female births only, produces the 'gross reproduction rate', which is typically about half of the total fertility rate.

If we were to allow our cohort of 1000 15-year-olds to die in each age group according to whatever death rates would be applicable for the age group, this clearly reduces the number of potential babies, and hence female babies. We derive the 'net reproduction rate' as the gross reproduction rate adjusted for relevant death rates of possible mothers.

Mortality Measures

The (crude) 'death rate' is defined rather like the crude birth rate, as the number of deaths per 1000 population in a period. The population is usually as estimated at mid year, from census data if available. The death rate is contingent on the age distribution of the population, and the ratio of males to females. The most convenient way to deal with this is to calculate 'age specific death rates', which are defined as the number of deaths in a particular age group in a period per 1000 population in that age group in the period. Separate calculations may be made for males and females to give sex–age specific rates.

An adjustment to the crude death rate can be made to take account of the varying proportion of old people in an area. An official government calculated 'area comparability' factor may be available for each geographical area. This factor takes into account the population structure of the preceding census, and by multiplying the crude death rate by the comparability factor it is possible to obtain a corrected death rate for use in comparisons.

The 'standardised death rate' can be used for general comparison on one population with another. In the direct method of calculation the age and sex compositions are deliberately standardised in the populations of interest to permit a valid comparison of deaths. When a standard population has been created, the particular age specific death rates for each country are applied to the standard population, to generate a hypothetical number of deaths. This number of deaths when expressed per 1000 population is the standardised death rate—in effect a kind of average death rate for the various age groups, but one which is obviously sensitive to the choice of 'standard population'.

A whole series of mortality rates exists dealing with specific groups, and we include a selection of the most important in the following sections.

The infant mortality rate is the number of deaths of infants under 1 year old in a period per 1000 live births in the period. Further analysis based on this rate may require information on whether the death is in the first seven days, the first 28 days or later. The 'early neonatal mortality rate' for a period is the number of deaths occurring within the first week of life per 1000 live births in the period. The 'neonatal mortality rate' is the number of deaths of infants under 28 days old per 1000 live births in the period, and the 'post neonatal mortality rate' is the number of deaths of infants aged 28 days and over per 1000 live births. Thus, the infant mortality rate is the sum of the neonatal and post neonatal mortality rates. The distinction between the two latter rates emphasises congenital factors in the first 28 days as against environmental factors later.

In all the infant related mortality rates the population at risk is defined as the number of live births, since stillbirths are not at risk of dying subsequently. The period usually used for the calculations is 1 year and, as it is usually a calendar year, some of the deaths reported within the calendar year really relate to births of the preceding year. And of course some births during the year will not result in a death until early in the following calendar year. In a fairly stable birth rate–mortality rate situation these marginal inaccuracies will not have much practical significance. If there are rapid changes in the birth rate, or if we are dealing with small numbers where small actual changes are large in percentage or 'rate' terms, then ideally the deaths should be related to the *relevant* live births.

Pregnancy does not always lead to a live birth even when we exclude spontaneous and planned abortions. In the final stages of pregnancy some babies still die and examination of the quality and efficiency of obstetric services requires recognition and measurements appertaining to these deaths. The definition of 'stillbirth' is not universal. In England the stillbirth is defined in the following way: 'A stillborn child is any child which has issued forth from the mother after the 28th week of pregnancy and which did not at any time after being completely expelled from the mother breathe or show any other sign of life.' The definition invites criticism which is outside the scope of this work. However, the difficulties of both deciding and reliably recording the occurrence of a stillbirth renders the calculation of the stillbirth rate less than wholly reliable. The 'stillbirth rate' is defined as the number of stillbirths in a period per 1000 births (live and still) in the period.

There is possibly some overlap of the stillbirth rate with the early neonatal mortality rate. Accordingly the 'perinatal mortality rate' includes both stillbirths and deaths within the first week, thus avoiding problems of distinguishing and/or recording correctly the time of death. The perinatal mortality rate is defined as the number of stillbirths and deaths occurring in the first week of life per 1000 births (live and still). The perinatal rate is widely used to assess the effectiveness of obstetric services.

The 'maternal mortality rate' is usually defined as the number of deaths of females attributed to childbirth per 1000 registered births (live and still). (Sometimes expressed as per 1000 *live* births.) Registered births are used as an approximation to pregnancies—which are not officially recorded—and the fact that multiple births can occur is ignored for the purposes of this calculation. The small numbers of maternal deaths in the UK has made this rate almost redundant.

Turning now to disease specific death, there are two rates to discuss. First, the 'disease specific mortality rate' is the number of persons dying of the disease in a period per 1000 population within which the deaths occurred. Second, the disease specific 'case fatality rate' is the number of persons dying of the disease in the period per 100 people who have the disease. Both 'rates' have the numerator as deaths attributable to the disease, but the denominators—reference populations—differ and, as pointed out earlier in this chapter, the case fatality 'rate' is really a ratio and is expressed per 100.

From the case fatality rate we can obtain 'standardised mortality ratios', which enable comparison of deaths from a particular disease over a period of time. Standardised mortality ratios are somewhat similar to standardised death rates which, it will be recalled, permit comparisons between countries despite different age and sex composition.

Suppose we know that for men the case fatality rate for disease X in 1975 is 2·5 per hundred. We will use 1975 as a 'base' year and obtain subsequent years fatality rates relative to 1975. Consider, for example, the year 1980, and suppose we apply the 2·5 per hundred 'rate' found in 1975 to the 1980 male population who contract the disease, say 50 000 people. The 1975 rate would predict 1250 deaths. If in fact we observed 1395 deaths, then this represents a worse situation than reflected by the 1975 rate, and we can obtain a 'relative' picture by computing the (SMR) 'standardised mortality ratio' as $1395/1250 \times 100 = 111{\cdot}6$. The definition of SMR is the ratio of actual deaths to expected deaths, multiplied by 100.

Morbidity Measures

Since few diseases are notifiable, our knowledge of morbidity is severely limited. The two principal morbidity measures are the incidence rate, which answers the question 'How many new cases?' and the prevalence rate, which answers 'How common is the disease?'.

The incidence rate for a disease is the number of new cases commencing in a specific period, per hundred of the population at risk. Incidence is the frequency of events during a period of time.

The (point) prevalence 'rate' is the number of cases of a particular disease existing in a population at a specified point in time, per hundred of the population at that time. Point prevalence is the census type of measure indicating 'how common' or how frequent a disease is at the point in time.

Incidence is a flow, concerned with new cases, whilst point prevalence is a stock, concerned with all existing cases. Point prevalence includes all persons having the disease irrespective of when it was contracted.

An alternative but less useful measure than the point prevalence is the period prevalence, which is the number of cases existing at any time within a specified period per 100 of the average population in the period. The period prevalence reflects the number of cases to be dealt with in the period, and is the sum of the point prevalence at the start of the period—i.e. the number of cases existing at the start—and the incidence rate in the period—i.e. the new cases reported during the period. Period prevalence is of limited use as we usually require to know whether cases are new or old, and thus the split into point prevalence and incidence is more useful. Indeed, the term 'prevalence' is usually used without specification as to 'point' or 'period', and when this is found it usually refers to point prevalence.

Sometimes when a disease is present in a community for only a short period, the incidence rate can be calculated after the short interval during which the disease is around, and even if the incidence rate was calculated at the usual time period of one year, it would not differ from that calculated at the end of the spate of illnesses. This special form of incidence rate for which there is a limited period of risk is called the 'attack rate'.

Life Tables

Suppose we follow through their lives a 'cohort' of 100 000 people born at a particular point in time and record how many die at each age. From such a 'longitudinal' cohort analysis we might produce, for example, the mean years of life experienced by a member of the group, or the mean number of future years available to a person of a given age. In practice we cannot find or follow 100 000 people born 'at a particular point in time' right through their lives. Instead we talk of a notional group and work out how many might die at each age if the age specific mortality rates currently known for each age are applied. These rates are used to assess how many persons of the 100 000 there would be in each succeeding year, producing the information in the life table, and in particular yielding the average future life expectation for a person of any age.

To simplify the arithmetic involved in a life table, let us consider a hypothetical population of creatures which never live to reach their sixth birthday, and suppose that 100 000 are born at a point in time and experience the age specific mortality rates shown in Table 32. The calculations begin as follows. The death rate in the first year of life, 300 per 1000, is applied to the 100 000 births and gives an expected 30 000 deaths during the year. The remaining 70 000 who enter their second year of life (beyond their first birthday) experience a death rate of 285·7 per 1000, which thus gives an expected 20 000 deaths. The remaining 50 000 who reach their second birthday experience a death rate of 400 per thousand resulting in 20 000 deaths, leaving 30 000 to reach their third birthday. Of these 333·3 per 1000 die leaving 20 000 to reach age 4. At age 4 the death rate is 500 per 1000, and thus 10 000 deaths occur between ages 4 and 5. This leaves 10 000 to reach their fifth birthday, where they experience a death rate of 1000 per 1000, and therefore no creatures reach age 6. The figures so far are shown in Table 33.

We now make a simplifying assumption that in any year the deaths occur in an evenly distributed manner during the year. Thus, in the first year of life there are 30 000 deaths and, on average, each creature which dies lives half a year. (In practice, of course, the neonatal mortality rate would usually indicate that deaths in the first year are predominantly in the very early part and 'real' life tables are adjusted for this.) Thus, a total of 30 000 × 0·5 years of life can be ascribed to those who die. Of course,

Table 32

Age Specific Mortality Rates for a Hypothetical Population

Age	Deaths Per 1000 Population
0	300
1	285·7
2	400
3	333·3
4	500
5	1 000

Table 33

Life Table Calculation—Stage 1: Annual Deaths Resulting from Applying Age Specific Mortality Rates to 100 000 Births

Age	Numbers Starting Year	Deaths in Year
0	100 000	30 000
1	70 000	20 000
2	50 000	20 000
3	30 000	10 000
4	20 000	10 000
5	10 000	10 000

70 000 survive the year and they 'assume' 70 000 years of life, making a grand total of $70\,000 + (30\,000 \times 0{\cdot}5) = 85\,000$ years of life 'lived' prior to age 1. Applying the same assumption to those who live beyond their first birthday, 20 000 die before age 2 and, thus, in this second year of life will between them accrue $20\,000 \times 0{\cdot}5$ years of life. A further 50 000 survive the full year, accruing 50 000 years during their second year of life, and we can now say that a total of $50\,000 + (20\,000 \times 0{\cdot}5)$ years of life are lived by the survivors in between their first and second birthdays. Table 34 shows the complete calculation at each stage. If we look ahead for the 100 000 from age 0 we see that together they enjoy a total of $85\,000 + 60\,000 + 40\,000 + 25\,000 + 15\,000 + 5000 = 230\,000$ years of

Table 34

Life Table Calculation—Stage 2: Calculation of Total (Combined) Years Lived in Each Year of Life

Age	Numbers Starting Year	Deaths in Year	Numbers Finishing Year	Total Years Lived in Year
0	100 000	30 000	70 000	$70\,000 + (30\,000 \times 0{\cdot}5) = 85\,000$
1	70 000	20 000	50 000	$50\,000 + (20\,000 \times 0{\cdot}5) = 60\,000$
2	50 000	20 000	30 000	$30\,000 + (20\,000 \times 0{\cdot}5) = 40\,000$
3	30 000	10 000	20 000	$20\,000 + (10\,000 \times 0{\cdot}5) = 25\,000$
4	20 000	10 000	10 000	$10\,000 + (10\,000 \times 0{\cdot}5) = 15\,000$
5	10 000	10 000	0	$0 + (10\,000 \times 0{\cdot}5) = 5\,000$

Table 35

Life Table Calculation—Stage 3: Calculation of (Combined) Years Lived in Each Year and Subsequently

Age	Numbers Starting Year	Years Lived in Year	Years Lived in Year and Subsequently
0	100 000	85 000	230 000
1	70 000	60 000	145 000
2	50 000	40 000	85 000
3	30 000	25 000	45 000
4	20 000	15 000	20 000
5	10 000	5 000	5 000

life. Therefore, the mean life expectation per member of this population is 230 000 ÷ 100 000 = 2·3 years.

Take as an example all who reach the age of 2. From Table 34 we see that 50 000 enter this age group, and live subsequent to the age of 2 a total of 40 000 + 25 000 + 15 000 + 5000 = 85 000 years. Therefore, per member of the population entering age group 2, there is on average 85 000 ÷ 50 000 = 1·7 years of further life to enjoy. We say that the mean expectation of life at age 2 is 1·7. To find the mean life expectation at each age we now add a further column to Table 34. This is the sum of the values in the 'total years lived in year' column at and beyond each age. At age 0, we already have a

Table 36

Life Table Calculation—Stage 4: Calculation of Mean Life Expectation at Each Age

Age	Mean Life Expectation
0	230 000 ÷ 10 000 = 2·30
1	145 000 ÷ 70 000 = 2·07
2	85 000 ÷ 50 000 = 1·70
3	45 000 ÷ 30 000 = 1·50
4	20 000 ÷ 20 000 = 1·00
5	5 000 ÷ 10 000 = 0·50

Table 37

Life Table for a Hypothetical Population

Age x	Numbers Starting Age x l_x	Deaths During Age x d_x	Total Years Lived During Age x L_x	Total Years Lived Beyond the Start of Age x T_x	Mean Life Expectancy of Those Who Start Age x e_x
0	100 000	30 000	85 000	230 000	2·30
1	70 000	20 000	60 000	145 000	2·07
2	50 000	20 000	40 000	85 000	1·70
3	30 000	10 000	25 000	45 000	1·50
4	20 000	10 000	15 000	20 000	1·00
5	10 000	10 000	5 000	5 000	0·50

future total of 230 000 years of life expectation by the starting cohort. At age 1 the sum of all the future years to be lived is 60 000 + 40 000 + 25 000 + 15 000 + 5000 = 145 000, and the figures for all the ages are made up and shown in Table 35.

The mean expectation of future life at each age is now calculated for each year by dividing 'years lived in year and subsequently' by number of 'entrants' to year, to give the final column shown in Table 36.

When we put together Tables 34, 35 and 36 into Table 37, we have the complete 'life table' for our hypothetical creature, and in each column of the table are indicated the usual symbols found in life tables.

A full detailed year by year life table for a human population

Table 38

A Life Table for Males and Females in the USA

Age Interval x	Number Starting Interval x l_x	Deaths in Age Interval x d_x	Mean Life Expectancy of Those Entering Interval x e_x
0–1	100 000	1 361	73·3
1–5	98 639	261	73·3
5–10	98 378	168	69·5
10–15	98 210	174	64·6
15–20	98 036	515	59·7
20–25	97 521	666	55·0
25–30	96 855	649	50·4
30–35	96 206	672	45·7
35–40	95 534	897	41·0
40–45	94 637	1 396	36·4
45–50	93 241	2 168	31·9
50–55	91 073	3 342	27·6
55–60	87 731	4 799	23·5
60–65	82 932	7 036	19·8
65–70	75 896	8 866	16·3
70–75	67 030	11 573	13·2
75–80	55 457	14 540	10·4
80–85	40 917	14 919	8·2
85	25 998	25 998	6·4

Source: National Center for Health Statistics, US Department of Health, Education and Welfare.

would start at age 0 and run up to around 110. To make the information easier to assimilate, it is usual to group ages as shown in the life table above (Table 38) and to suppress some of the columns, leaving only the most important. In effect, it is as though each age, x, dealt with in Table 37 has become an 'interval' x in Table 38.

Separate life tables can be constructed for particular groups, such as males/females; socioeconomic groups; occupational groups; and looking at people who contract a disease they can be followed in much the same way as the life table follows a cohort of births to give prognoses of future life at any period after the reported contraction of the disease. Similarly, the concept of the life table has been applied to hospital inpatient populations, especially psychiatric hospitals, regarding time spent in hospital as an age, and thus working with 'hospital age' rather than physical age.

Life tables are extremely useful in making comparisons between populations. Perhaps the most important disadvantage is that it is calculated on rates applicable at a particular point in time. As a real cohort moves forward, the true applicable rates will be different. Nevertheless, as a guide to where significant reductions in mortality are happening, and as a pointer to where future effort is required, the life table is a valuable indicator in community medicine. A final cautionary note: life tables relate to large numbers of people. They do not tell anything about a particular person, and do not indicate variability from person to person.

10

Bed Utilisation Statistics

Introduction

Hospital doctors who function as members of management teams need an understanding of resource utilisation measures. Four of the most useful indexes relating to the utilisation of beds are the average length of a patient's stay in a bed; the average time a bed remains empty between patients, known as the 'turnover interval'; the percentage of beds, on average, occupied; and the separations per available bed, known as 'throughput'. This chapter provides a brief resume of these utilisation measures.

Average (Mean) Length of Stay

The average length of stay is the mean number of days spent continuously in hospital by a typical patient. There are two approaches to calculating this statistic. The first is to record the number of days of stay of each patient, and then to calculate the mean. If it is seen that one or two patients are, through extremely long stays, distorting the mean, then the median is a possible but little-used alternative. The advantage of the method of recording each individual patient's length of stay is that the standard deviation of the length of stay can be calculated at the same time as the mean, and can then be used to indicate the uniformity or variability from patient to patient, which is of course just as important as the average. Recording systems in current use ensure that the mean length of stay is *not* normally calculated in the way just described. Instead it is usual to add the daily number of occupied beds for a month, and divide that by the number of patients who 'separate' from those beds in the same period. 'Separation' includes transfers, discharges and deaths.

Suppose that for a particular ward in June the number of occupied and available beds at a stated time on each day have been as shown in Table 39. There have been 50 'separations' from the ward recorded in the month. The usual method of obtaining average (mean) length of stay is to work out how many bed-days have been utilised in this period and to allocate these to the 50

Table 39

Bed Availability in the Month of June

Date	Beds Occupied	Available Beds
1	20	25
2	21	25
3	20	25
4	22	25
5	22	25
6	22	25
7	21	25
8	22	26
9	19	26
10	18	26
11	18	26
12	19	26
13	20	26
14	21	26
15	22	26
16	18	26
17	17	26
18	19	26
19	19	26
20	18	26
21	19	26
22	20	26
23	20	25
24	20	25
25	19	25
26	18	24
27	20	24
28	21	24
29	19	24
30	20	24
Totals	594	760

patients who have separated, on the assumption that these patients are typical. The figure for bed-days used up is obtained by adding together the figures in the 'occupied beds' column of Table 39, i.e. 20 + 21 + 20 + ... + 19 + 20 = 594 days (this is a total bed-use figure for the month). Dividing by 50 we obtain 11·88 days; the average length of stay per patient. Therefore, if returns on bed state are available routinely and numbers of separations similarly, then the calculation is easily made.

It should be noted that the 50 separations have themselves not occupied the beds for the 50 bed-days. Some of these separations will in fact leave in the first few days of the month, and some of the occupied days, especially at the end, will be provided by patients who do not 'separate' in the month and are therefore not in the separations figure. Thus, it is true that the 594 bed-days are not 'personal' to the particular 50 patients who separate. We therefore need to be satisfied that we are looking at a long enough period for the 50 separations to be *typical* and a steady state to exist, so that if we were to go to the trouble of getting the correct 50 patients, they would be little or no different to the 50 actually used. The period we consider then must be of substantial length; preferably at least five or six times the average length of stay. This way we are unlikely to have a patient who is hospitalised right through the period without leaving, because such a patient would distort our statistics. He would contribute bed-days, but now allow a corresponding separation to be recorded.

The alternative method, which is slower and more demanding, yet accurate and indicative of variability, is to record the exact

Table 40

Completed Days of Hospital Stay for 50 Separations in a Month

14	12	9	11	12
7	11	17	2	13
12	14	9	13	12
13	9	13	9	11
11	12	21	7	9
12	13	14	19	10
9	9	9	11	11
15	18	11	11	13
6	7	12	11	14
11	8	11	12	20

number of days of stay of each of the 50 leavers in the month. Suppose these are as in Table 40. From these data we can calculate the exact mean stay length as 11·6 days and, most importantly, the standard deviation of this length stay, which works out as 3·44 days.† We then have the beginnings of a monitoring tool which can be regularly updated, indicating the level and its variation from patient to patient, and the consistency of behaviour of the medical staff. Notice that the exact mean (11·6 days) is slightly different, as would be expected, from the previous mean of 11·88 days, which was of course an estimate based on the 50 leavers.

The Turnover Interval

The mean time between a patient leaving a bed and a new patient entering is known as the turnover interval. Obviously efficient resource utilisation requires this to be minimised, and achievement of a low turnover interval would improve bed occupancy. The turnover interval gives an indication of the efficiency of admission procedures. Each time a patient separates from the ward or unit, the number of complete days for which the bed is empty could be recorded. For the 50 separations of Table 40, we should have 50 figures listing the empty bed-days. It is then possible to calculate, for the 50, the mean and standard deviation. This mean is the true turnover interval.

The usual method used is different from this being based on bed state figures, and precludes us from obtaining a measure of variability such as the standard deviation. It is, however, computationally quite simple. We first add together the number of occupied beds in Table 39 for each of the 30 days, to get the occupied bed-days in the ward that month. This sum is 594 days. Next we add the available bed-days for each of the 30 days to get the total available days, which comes to 760.

The difference between these figures, 166 days, represents empty-bed-days, and spread over the 50 separations gives a mean of 3·32 days per separation. Thus, the turnover interval is recorded as 3·32 days.

† The standard deviation has been calculated using the 'n' method because here it is being employed as a descriptive statistic and no sample inferences are sought. The 'n' method is used throughout this chapter.

Percentage Bed Occupancy

The mean percentage bed occupancy derives from the same figures as turnover interval. It is usually calculated by noting that in our example of the 760 available bed-days, 594 were utilised giving a mean percentage occupancy of $(594/760) \times 100 = 78{\cdot}2\%$. Unfortunately, the variations in occupancy are probably more important than the mean percentage level, and this usual approach does not permit their assessment.

If instead we were to derive from Table 39 the *daily* percentage occupancy, and thus work with 30 such figures, we could calculate the mean *and* standard deviation. The daily percentage occupancy for day 1 is $(20/25) \times 100 = 80\%$, and Table 41 lists the comparable figures for each day of the month. The overall mean is 78·2% as before, but we now have the standard deviation of 6·4% as our second statistic, which enables valid month-to-month comparisons for this ward, and within-month comparisons of this ward with others.

Table 41

Daily Percentage Bed Occupancy

Date	Percentage Occupancy	Date	Percentage Occupancy
1	80	16	69·2
2	84	17	65·4
3	80	18	73·1
4	88	19	73·1
5	88	20	69·2
6	88	21	73·1
7	84	22	76·9
8	84·6	23	80
9	73·1	24	80
10	69·2	25	76
11	69·2	26	75
12	73·1	27	83·3
13	76·9	28	87·5
14	80·8	29	79·2
15	84·6	30	83·3

Throughput

The throughput of a ward is the number of separations (discharges, deaths and transfers) divided by the mean number of available beds. In our example we have 50 discharges in the month. The mean number of available beds is obtained by adding the figures in the 'available beds' column of Table 39 to obtain 760 and dividing by 30 to give 25·3. The throughput is then 50 for 25·3 beds, which is 50/25·3 per bed, i.e. 1·97 per bed. Clearly shorter lengths of stay can produce higher throughputs per bed, and this can be reinforced by a small turnover interval. It is well known that the statistics of bed utilisation are interlinked—high throughput would suggest, for example, a low turnover interval, high average occupancy and short average stay. The interdependence of the bed utilisation measures can be presented graphically and is discussed by Barber and Johnson (1973), by Tyrrell (1975) and by Yates (1983).

References

Barber B. and Johnson D. (1973). The presentation of acute hospital in-patient statistics. *Hospital & Health Services Review*; **69**(1): 11–14.

Cottrell K.M. (1980). Waiting lists: Some problems of definition and a relative measure of waiting time. *Hospital & Health Services Review*; **78**(8): 265–74.

Tyrrell M. (1975). *Using Numbers for Effective Health Service Management.* London: Heinemann.

Yates J. (1983). *Hospital Beds.* London: Heinemann.

11

Computers

Introduction

In future years the computer may well become as indispensable as the stethoscope to many types of doctor. The mystique surrounding the computer, reinforced as it is by 'computer jargon' will need to be stripped away as more and more computers will be available for use. It is likely that in the not-too-distant future the 'home' computer will be as common as the domestic television; children will operate computers at home and at school; and future patients will be familiar with computer practice and expect, for example, to have computerised diagnostics, or computer based medical records.

Speculation aside, even if the above suggestions are wrong, the 'computer' has many benefits to confer on medicine, not least of which is the simplification of complex statistical work. Doctors with only a basic understanding of statistics will be able, indeed some currently are able, to command and observe the instantaneous execution of statistical routines that would have taken armies of statisticians weeks or months to carry out.

Computers and Some Jargon

A computer is a machine which can execute arithmetic and logical operations at speeds millions of times greater than the human brain. Computers add, subtract, and by the process of repeated addition or repeated subtraction they can multiply or divide. Computers can also compare two numbers, which we may call A and B, and recognise which, if either, is the greater. They can then act 'logically' according to this discovery, executing tasks appropriate to the possible situations: A exceeds B; or A equals B; or A is less than B. Computers are available in two main types: the analogue and the digital. The former represent numbers by actual physical quantities, such as electrical voltages. The simplest type of analogue 'computer' is a slide rule, which uses physical lengths to represent numbers. Digital computers represent numerical quantities by discrete electrical states which can be altered to represent arithmetic quantities. Most medical and health care administrative use of computers is dependent on the digital type.

Computers work basically in the following manner. They can command data to be transmitted as an input from a 'peripheral device', such as a 'card reader'. They can then analyse the data, perform mathematical and logical operations on it, combine it with different data, make logical decisions, and command a peripheral device to transmit the results either into a readable form, or onto some storage medium. In order to command input, compute, and provide output the computer has a 'memory', a 'control unit' (which directs the computer's operations), and an arithmetic unit. The memory has to store the 'program', which is a step by step guide to the computer to exactly what operations it must do. The memory also will hold data and calculations in progress. The control unit, the memory (or 'storage unit') and the arithmetic unit make up the 'central processing unit'. The peripheral devices which can provide the central processing unit with input data are machines such as card readers, tape drives, disc drives and light-sensitive pens which are applied to television type screens. The peripherals which are used to transmit output are items such as cathode ray tubes which give a television-like display, line printers which type out results, magnetic tape units which record results on tape, graph plotters, etc.

In a manual data handling system, a clerk operates with a procedures handbook, some of which he remembers, some not. Suppose he is asked to review a waiting list for gastro-intestinal surgery and bring to the surgeon's attention cases waiting more than a specified time, say six months, or cases in certain age groups. He will establish some kind of 'search procedure', perhaps first pulling out all the records of patients who have waited six months or more, then extracting from those left patients over 65, and then sorting the total of those extracted into one of two categories: over 65, waiting six months or more; under 65, waiting six months or more. The pre-established 'search and report' sequence of operations is a program for action analogous to a computer program. This program is stored in the clerk's memory, which is analogous to the computer memory. He himself acts as the 'processor' of the information. He then provides a typed report, analogous to the computer output of a list of names.

The physical equipment which goes to make up a computer is referred to as 'hardware'. For a microcomputer the basic hardware is about the size of a small portable television set.

The main internal memory of modern computers is often called 'core memory' because it is made up from stacks of small ferrite rings called 'cores'. Cores are very easily magnetised, and are strung like beads on a wire. When a current is passed through the wire the cores are magnetised in the direction of the flow of the current. Reversing the flow will reverse the magnetism. Thus, two different 'states' can be experienced by a magnetised core, and these can represent binary numbers 0 and 1. All numbers can be 'built up' in the binary system based on 0 and 1, and thus arithmetic can be carried out by magnetising cores.

Core memory is expensive and so the computer will usually have additionally auxiliary memory in the form of external storage, and will be able to transmit data to and receive data from these external sources, which are usually magnetic discs, drums or tape.

In large-scale systems a popular form of storage (to the computers the analogy for paper files and storage filing cabinet) is the punched card. A data file consists of a set of punched cards. The 'IBM' card has 80 columns and 12 rows. Data are entered using a machine called a 'keypunch'. Each letter or number punched appears both as a set of holes, and in typewritten form at the top of the card. Whilst cheap and convenient for manual handling, punched cards are easily damaged, may get out of order, and cannot be amended. When a change is required, a new card must be punched. They are also 'slow', in-so-far as 'reading' them by the computer, or transferring data onto them. In effect, the punched card is obsolete except for small jobs, and in its place we have a variety of possibilities: magnetic tape, disks, and drums on which data are represented by magnetising certain areas. Data amendment can be carried out by first demagnetising and then remagnetising the relevant section.

The magnetic tape is a compact way of storing large quantities of data, which cannot become mixed up. The machine which both reads and prepares a tape is called a 'tape drive'. There is usually a tape drive for reading in data, and a separate tape drive for writing a tape as output from the computer.

A magnetic tape cannot be read by people in the way that punched cards can. A computer has to read a tape and make any changes necessary. Magnetic tape storage systems require the computer to read the complete contents of a file up to the desired section. This method of access is called serial access. When the storage system allows access directly to the relevant part of the file without running right through all the records in it, we describe it as having random access. Magnetic tape is not a random access system, and would not be used where speed of information flow is important.

A tape storage system is good for large files when we are able to treat each in the same simple systematic way for sorting, amending, checking, etc., without requesting random access, or quick access to a particular patient's records.

To get over the problem of serial access to magnetic tape, there are several types of equipment available, the most common being 'magnetic disks' and 'magnetic drums'. The method of recording is to place magnetised spots on the disk or drum. These spots can contain a great deal of information, and the computer can access them almost instantly, knowing where each spot is and what it contains. When it is important, as in dealing with medical records, to extract random items of information in a file, the disk or drum storage method—called 'mass storage'—offers major gains in efficiency over magnetic tape.

'Software' relates to non-hardware items in a computer system. Software therefore includes the programs which serve to make the computer system carry out its tasks. To actually control the way the computer operates there are special programs called 'system software'.

The 'languages' in which programs are written are not usually those in which the computer operates. Many currently available languages such as BASIC—beginner's all-purpose symbolic instruction code—and COBOL—common business oriented language—are so similar to everyday English that no prior programming experience is required to learn to write in a short period (a few days at most) programs ranging from those for biochemical analysis to programs for keeping accounts in a general practice. The computer is equipped with programs called 'compilers' which convert these 'high level' languages into instructions which the machines can follow.

Many computer systems are equipped with 'software libraries', which include 'suites' of statistical programs. These are often referred to as 'canned' programs or 'packages'.

Statistical Packages

Statistical 'packages' are in increasing use by statisticians, medical researchers, social researchers, and a wide variety of others ranging from geographers to cryptanalysts. The names of these packages are usually abbreviated. For example, SAS means Statistical Analysis System, and SPSS is Statistical Package for the Social Sciences. Despite the 'social' in its title, SPSS is in wide use in medical studies and is quite typical of these 'packages'. SPSS is an integrated system of computer programs designed for the analysis of data. In one easy to use system it provides all the tools needed for statistical analysis. People who use a statistical package need methods for information storage and retrieval, for modification and for requesting specific statistical analyses, for report writing, and for combining observations for several data sets, with appropriate editing, merging and updating procedures. Statistical packages have all these facilities.

The actual statistical capabilities of these packages are extensive. As long as the user can gain access for himself and his data to a computer system which boasts, for example SPSS, then he has at his fingertips procedures ranging from simple descriptive statistics, such as means and standard deviations, histograms, and cross tabulations to correlation and regression analyses, statistical tests, analysis of variance, discriminant analysis, factor analysis, etc., etc. In addition, 'packages' can create 'new' variables, modify variables, and re-arrange and sort data. For example, in a large-scale health survey in which responses arrive randomly from people in different cities, they may be input to the computer as they arrive. The program can then, when it is desired, put the data into order by city population size, and then within each city by the names of people alphabetically for any subgroup, and go on to obtain descriptive statistics, draw histograms, scatter diagrams, make cross tabulations, and so on.

SPSS and similar packages are driven through their various

functions by a sequence of 'control' instructions, prepared in a highly specific manner. The data for SPSS is usually punched onto 80 column IBM cards, or entered into the computer via a terminal in an equivalent way. The data are organised into 'files'. A file consists of the user's data and associated information entered on the 'control' cards, describing and defining the data. Before it can interpret and analyse any data, the computer needs a name for the data file, a list of variables that are included, the fact that the information is on, say, cards, the location of the variables on the punched cards, and the number of cases covered by the data. Typically, cards would be prepared containing words as follows: FILENAME; VARIABLE LIST; INPUT MEDIUM CARD; INPUT FORMAT; NUMBER OF CASES. The point of including these names in this book is to indicate that the preparation of the instructions to the computer is simple and logical; it is told in the clearest manner exactly what is being offered to it, and subsequently what procedures to carry out.

Variables are frequently entered in some coded manner. For example, sex may be entered as the first variable and called variable number 1. Age may be variable number 2, and principal diagnosis number 3. When the computer prints out results it will use 1, 2, 3 and so on unless it is told the correct names of the variables. A card called VAR LABELS, short for variable labels, instructs the computer that variable 1, when printed at the end of the computer run should be printed as 'sex', variable 2 as 'age' and variable 3 as 'principal diagnosis'.

The values or categories *within* any variable may also be coded. Sex has categories 'male' and 'female', which we might enter into the computer under codes 0 and 1. Age group may have values 15–24, 25–34, 35–44, etc., which we might code 0, 1, 2, etc. When a printout of results is obtained, it is much more readable if the computer prints 'male' instead of '0', and 'female' instead of 1. Accordingly, a card called VALUE LABELS instructs the computer to print a particular label, such as 'male' wherever a particular code value, such as 0, appears within the sex variable. Sometimes in a study, for a variety of reasons, data are not recorded. Personnel are often too busy to record data at the relevant time and a questionnaire has 'blanks' when it is received for analysis. The computer would be told this on a MISSING VALUES card.

Once the data has been described fully as above, there follow a series of cards such as 'CROSSTABS' which will carry out a cross tabulation of any specified variables, such as diagnosis by sex; 'FREQUENCIES', which will provide a frequency distribution, print out a histogram, supply means, medians, modes, standard deviations and so on; REGRESSION, which will carry out regression analysis; T-TEST, which performs *t* tests, etc., etc.

When the control cards described above are complete, then the data cards need preparation. Suppose a survey of 20 people records the name, sex, age, weight and height. A *data value* is a single measurement, such as Mr. Jones' *age*. An observation is an associated set of data values, such as Mr. Jones' *name*, *age*, *sex*, *height* and *weight*.

The measurements on, for example, the weights of all 20 people make up the weight *variable*. The other variables are formed similarly. A variable is a set of data values for the same measurement, such as the number of calories for each packet of a particular food, or the humidity level day by day in a room.

Most collections of data are made up of many observations. Each observation contains several data values. These collections of data are called 'data sets'. The values in Table 42 are a data set. The values on each line are an observation. Within each observation, any single value, say C's age, 71, is a data value. The first value in observation is the name, which is an *alphabetic character* or a 'character' variable. The other values are numbers, and called 'numeric'.

To get the data into a form the computer can read they might be punched onto cards. Each card has 80 columns and each individual from A to T has his or her own card. Where there is a great deal of information per person, a second or more cards can be used. In the case of the data set in Table 42 we might proceed as follows: In column 1 of a card we punch the name, in column 2 the sex, in columns 3, 4 and 5 the age (allowing three columns because of the possibility of someone over 100 turning up later); in columns 6, 7 and 8 the weight, and in columns 9 and 10 the height. In columns 3, 4 and 5, if we were dealing with someone aged 9, the values punched would be 009.

Once the data are fully punched and carefully checked, then the control cards and the data can be submitted to the computer as a 'job'. Provided there are no errors in the specifications or punching, the output will be generated automatically, usually typed out at high speed on a line-printer.

Table 42

A Data Set

Name	Sex	Age (years)	Weight (lb)	Height (in)
A	F	46	150	66
B	M	32	180	72
C	F	71	101	60
D	F	45	112	62
E	M	33	116	70
F	M	29	170	69
G	M	42	184	68
H	F	49	121	63
I	M	51	169	67
J	M	46	160	76
K	F	74	91	59
L	F	39	124	63
M	F	44	139	64
N	M	55	171	69
O	F	63	145	65
P	F	46	137	64
Q	F	62	118	61
R	M	49	194	70
S	F	28	117	64
T	F	19	130	66

```
BEANB                                                        23/12/80      18.17.55.    PAGE  16

FILE   GOLD       (CREATION DATE  =  23/12/80 )

VAR009

       CODE
            I
        2.  ********* (      3)
            I
            I
        3.  ************************** (      10)
            I
            I
        4.  ******************************************************** (      20)
            I
            I
        9.  *********** (      4)
(MISSING)   I
            I
            I.........I.........I.........I.........I.........I
                      4         8        12        16        20
            FREQUENCY

MEAN            3.515      STD ERR          .116      MEDIAN          3.675
MODE            4.000      STD DEV          .667      VARIANCE         .445
KURTOSIS         .050      SKEWNESS       -1.067      RANGE           2.000
MINIMUM         2.000      MAXIMUM         4.000      SUM           116.000
C.V. PCT       18.979      .95 C.I.        3.279          T           3.752

VALID CASES        33      MISSING CASES      4
```

Fig. 28. Simulated printout from an SPSS 'package'.

Figure 28 shows some descriptive statistics produced by an SPSS program in the course of a study on the efficiency of a 'bead' bed, which is designed to reduce the incidence of pressure lesions in hospital patients (Goldstone *et al.*, 1982). The study looked at elderly patients in orthopaedic wards. Variable 009 is blood pressure, which was coded according to its level on a scale 1 to 4 inclusive. Code 9 indicates a missing value. There were 33 cases in which the blood pressure was recorded, and four in which it was omitted. The computer has printed out a 'histogram' made up from asterisks, with an obvious mode at level 4.

From another part of the same study, Fig. 29 shows the analysis of size of broken skin in a 'control' group of patients who were not treated using the bead bed, but rather received the orthodox mattress and aids. Variable 145 is the maximum diameter in millimetres of broken skin on the sacrum postoperatively during hospitalisation. The computer has indicated a number of statistics including a mean of 81·111, a standard deviation of 51·404, a minimum of 5·000 and a maximum of 150·000. In particular, it has counted nine valid cases (who contracted a pressure lesion) and 28 missing cases, who remained free of sores. Notice that variable 009, the blood pressure, was *categorised* for recording purposes, but in contrast variable 145 is the actual magnitude in millimetres. Packages such as SPSS can handle both categorical variables and actual values of variables.

Non-statistical Use of Computers in Medicine

Computers can be programmed to simulate systems and predict the consequences of change within those systems. A 'model' of a system is fed into the computer, which can then printout the possible consequences of change in a parameter of the model. For example, the growth of an epidemic can be simulated, and the consequence of random populations movements can be assessed, or the consequence of a shift in the infection rate can be studied. A factor which promotes a simulation approach is that the elements of a system should be random, so that many possible results could ensue. Epidemics involve random contraction by people of the infection. Admissions to a psychiatric hospital in any year is likely to be a random number. Retentions beyond any period of patients within the hospital is a chance situation. And discharges from the

VARIABLE VAR 145								
MEAN	81·111	STD ERR	17·135	STD DEV	51·404	24/12/80	09/58/45	Page 150
VARIANCE	2642·361	KURTOSIS	−1·102	SKEWNESS	−·293			
MINIMUM	5·000	MAXIMUM	150·000	SUM	730·000			
C.V. PCT	63·375	·95 C.I.	41·599	TO	120·624			
VALID CASES	9	MISSING CASES	28					

Fig. 29. Simulated printout from an SPSS 'package'.

existing 'stock' of patients also has a random element. Consequently, prediction of patient numbers for the future is very much a guessing game. By simulating various possibilities a computer approach can systematise the guesswork and see how sensitive future numbers are to particular factors or parameters.

Simulation is also possible for the working of physiological systems such as heart, lungs, blood chemistry, etc. Computer simulation in diagnosis can avoid costly mistakes. A hypothetical patient can be programmed into the computer, along with responses to potential questions that a medical student may put. Even reactions to treatment can be included. The medical student can thus safely and cheaply diagnose and treat his computer patient. The output from the diagnosis might even be a list of possibles, in decreasing order of probability.

In real diagnostic situations the computer may be used for preliminary questions. This can be particularly helpful where sensitive or embarrassing question content is involved. People may feel happier responding to computer 'probes'. Systems exist in which the patient answers the computer merely by touching the appropriate response on a screen with a light sensitive pen. Cartoon type question and response systems also are in use to take patients through preliminary medical interviews, and produce a printout of medical history prior to the real consultation. A major benefit from computer-assisted diagnosis is that the collective wisdom of many specialists can be 'automated' into the system, giving the responsible doctor a first class up-to-date back up.

The list of computer applications in direct and indirect patient care is long. Computers can monitor equipment relating to a patient's blood pressure, respiration rate, heart rate, body temperature, cardiac output, venous pressure, urine output..., providing printed records and sounding off warnings as appropriate. Computers can clarify interpretations of x-rays, signal abnormalities and prepare lists of likely causes in rank order of probability. Clinical laboratories are the heaviest, non-administrative medical users of computers. Pathology, especially haematology and biochemistry, is a main user.

The data processing capability of the computer can be used in screening, where large numbers of people undergo routine comprehensive examinations by doctors. Computers deal well with this type of high volume detailed information, and they can be programmed to collate test results for individuals and print 'personal' reports, as well as compute overall population statistics.

Medical record linkage is a particularly useful capability of computers. Record linkage is the inclusion of a time dimension into a patient's medical records that the main medical events in his history such as birth, hospitalisation, and death are easily traceable. Detailed medical case notes are not the input to record linkage systems. Instead, only the major features are inputs, such as diagnoses, operations, length of hospital stay, accidents, and drug sensitivities. This kind of information is usually already collected within health care systems which do not have computer based systems. The computer aspect requires a re-organisation of the data processing function to link the information through time. Thus, through record linkage later events can be related to earlier ones, cohorts can be followed, long-term effects can be monitored, genetic change can become observable, etc., etc. The popular form of study made possible is the longitudinal study—a follow up of patients over a period of time.

Medical administrative uses of the computer are many and varied: community health registers and recall systems; appointment systems; patient scheduling; management of waiting lists; bed state management; nurse allocation and deployment; menu planning; personnel information systems; patient medical and nursing records; pharmaceutical systems for ordering and controlling drug stocks; radiology reporting and record retrieval; health administration statistics such as hospital activity analysis; hospital laboratory quality control systems . . . the list is continually lengthening. The computer has undoubtedly become a major tool pervading many aspects of health care and its management and research. One problem which has not yet been solved is the problem that the computer can give too much. It is common for an excess of information to be requested, beyond that which can be digested by the user. The result frequently is a paper mountain. The computer, if possible, should be used in a discriminating manner, and not requested to report and print every mundane statistic. It is useful if pre-set limits can be set for variables, such that when data lie within these limits, the data are accepted as 'normal' and no printout results. This is an example of reporting by exception.

Another problem is of the tail wagging the dog. The computer programmers in any system need to write programs to satisfy clinical or administrative requirements. Because of their intimate knowledge of computers and computing and the jargon they use, it is all too easy for computer personnel to over-influence the output they provide.

Conclusions

The computer will probably do at least as much to change the nature and future of the world as the wheel or the printing press. Everyone is affected by computers, and everyone is a statistic residing in the memory of one of these machines.

The computer is a tool which makes possible the multiplication of the capabilities of the human brain by millions. At present computers run telephone exchanges, prepare weather forecasts, 'compose' music, 'run' commercial banking systems, run hotel reservation systems, plan menus, schedule appointments . . . the list is long and ever increasing.

Computers can store vast amounts of information and give almost instant recall. They can calculate in seconds problems which would take centuries for people to solve. In short, computers represent a most powerful tool for the scientist, technologist, administrator and doctor. It is essential that today's and tomorrow's doctor take advantage of this tool, which may well become as indispensable as the stethoscope. Computers will become more and more part of life, as common as the domestic television. In only a very few years most general practitioners will be ill-equipped unless they can boast at least a micro computer.

Computers are incredibly fast, but they do not think and are not creative. They can only follow immaculately the instructions given to them in a program. In terms of intelligence, they have no more than an auroscope, which is useless without a guiding hand and an interpretive eye. Computers manipulate and process data. They cannot spontaneously make decisions. The only decisions they may make must be pre-programmed in terms of simple logical conditions.

A computer is instructed by a person via a computer program to carry out logical and arithmetical operations. The computer is no more than an electronic servant. It cannot make ethical judgements, nor moral decisions, nor exercise discretion or wisdom. This servant is becoming cheaper to purchase, and physically of a more convenient size all the time. The micro computer has the potential to revolutionise aspects of medical practice, ranging from general practice, where it can schedule appointments, help in diagnostics and handle patients' records, to complex medical scientific work. 'Conversational' computing, in which the user types in commands to the computer and receives almost instant response, has made computing easier to learn, and of wide applicability where immediate results are required. The processing of the user's work is done almost immediately, and is referred to as in 'real time' processing, without delays of having to submit a job and wait perhaps hours or overnight for the results, as in 'batch processing'. A large ('mainframe') computer equipped with many physically remote terminals can handle the work of many users apparently simultaneously. Each person has direct 'on-line' access to the computer. Each user appears to get instant response, although in fact he is served on a cycle with occasional brief delays. In the not-too-distant future it will be an entirely reasonable expectation for every doctor to have either a computer terminal in his office linked to a remote computer or a micro computer for his personal use.

Reference

Goldstone L.A., Norris M., O'Reilly M. and Whyte J. (1982). A clinical trial of a bead bed system for the prevention of pressure sores in elderly orthopaedic patients. *J. Adv. Nurse;* **7**:545–8.

Appendix 1: Further Reading

A. Introductory, General and Medical Statistics Books Using a Narrative Style

Brodie M. (1972). *On Thinking Statistically*. London: Heinemann.
Castle W.M. (1979). *Statistics in Operation*. Edinburgh: Churchill Livingstone.
Huff D. (1954). *How to Lie with Statistics*. London: Gollancz. Republished. (1973). Harmondsworth: Penguin Books.
Tanur J.M. (1972). *Statistics: A Guide to the Unknown*. San Francisco: Holden-Day.
Tippett L.A.C. (1968). *Statistics*. Oxford University Paperbacks.
Wallis W.A. and Roberts H.V. (1962). *The Nature of Statistics*. New York: The Free Press.
Wheeler M. (1976). *Lies, Damn Lies, and Statistics*. New York: Liveright.

B. Introductory Textbooks Using Mainly Narrative Style

Bailey N.T.J. (1959). *Statistical Methods in Biology*. London: English Universities Press.
Bourke G.J. and McGilvray J. (1975). *Interpretation and Uses of Medical Statistics*. 2nd edition. Oxford: Blackwell.
Goldstone L.A. (1980). *Statistics in the Management of Nursing Services*. London: Pitman Medical.
Hill A.B. (1977). *A Short Textbook of Medical Statistics*. London: Unibooks, Hodder and Stoughton.
Kilpatrick S.J. (1977). *Statistical Principles in Health Care Information*. Baltimore: University Park Press.
Mainland D. (1963). *Elementary Medical Statistics*. Philadelphia: W.B. Saunders.

C. Textbooks, and Textbook-style Work Books Using Symbolic Notation

Bahn A.K. (1972). *Basic Medical Statistics.* New York: Grune and Stratton.
Castle W.M. (1977). *Statistics in Small Doses.* 2nd edition. Edinburgh: Churchill Livingstone.
Harper W.M. (1977). *Statistics.* 3rd edition. M and E Handbooks Series. London: Macdonald and Evans.
Hammerton M. (1975). *Statistics for the Human Sciences.* London and New York: Longman.
Petrie A. (1978). *Lecture Notes on Medical Statistics.* Oxford: Blackwell.
Swinscow T.D.V. (1977). *Statistics at Square One.* 2nd edition. London: British Medical Association.
Von Fraunhofer J.A. and Murray J.J. (1981). *Statistics in Medical, Dental and Biological Studies.* London: Tri-Med Books.

D. Books on Special Topics and Research

Armitage P. (1973). *Statistical Methods in Medical Research,* 2nd edition. Oxford: Blackwell.
Armitage P. (1975). *Sequential Medical Trials.* Oxford: Blackwell.
Benjamin B. (1968). *Health and Vital Statistics.* London: George Allen and Unwin.
England J.M. (1975). *Medical Research, a Statistical and Epidemiological Approach.* Edinburgh: Churchill Livingstone.
Federer W. (1973). *Statistics and Society: Data Collection and Interpretation.* New York: Marcel Dekker.
Moser C.A. and Kalton G. (1972). *Survey Methods in Social Investigation.* London: Heinemann.
Osborn J.F. (1978). *Statistical Exercises in Medical Research.* Oxford: Blackwell.
Tyrrell M. (1975). *Using Numbers for Effective Health Service Management.* London: Heinemann.
Raj D. (1972). *The Design of Sample Surveys.* New York: McGraw-Hill.

Appendix 2: Probability

Introduction

Imagine a situation where there are four possible diagnoses, and only one can be correct. Suppose you make the choice of one, knowing that all four are equally likely. We would say that the probability of making the correct choice is 1/4.

Suppose 100 of a particular organ transplant in fairly similar circumstances have been attempted in the past, and the number of successful operations—according to some predetermined criterion—is 10. The probability of a successful transplant is then $10/100 = 1/10$.

The traditional definition of probability is the number of times an event has occurred divided by the number of opportunities to occur that it had. This definition looks at the relative frequency of occurrence and is a historical approach.

Sometimes we do not have any historical precedent for the event we are considering. When the first kidney transplant was carried out, the reply to the question 'What is the probability of success?' could not come from looking at the history of the operations. Yet the team conducting the surgery must have had some scientific or intuitive feelings that there was a good or reasonable chance of success. In other words, it might have been possible for the surgeons to say: we believe we have a 50% chance of success, or, we believe we have a probability of success equal to 1/2. Where does such a probability come from? Clearly not historical experience. All we can say is that it reflects the legitimate intensity of belief of the team. In other words, some probabilities are subjective. Suppose as the operation is being carried out the confidence of the team increases and the prognosis looks better than at the start.

They may well feel that the probability of success is higher than at first estimated, say 60%, or 0·6. The probability is thus revised. As long as we accept that probability reflects strength of belief, then it is possible to update a probability in the light of new information. Obviously the maximum value of a probability is 1, representing certainty that the outcome will occur. The minimum is 0, indicating that it will definitely not occur. When we deal with an uncertain situation in which there are several possible outcomes, each with several alternative consequences, the concept of probability can help to clarify the thought processes necessary prior to the situation. In particular, there are ways of combining probabilities of separate elements in a complex series of events so that a realistic assessment can be made of the total situation.

For example, suppose there is a probability of 0·9 that a consultant has made a correct diagnosis of a patient's condition. The patient is then referred elsewhere to a clinic where there is a probability of 0·7 that he gets the correct treatment as originally prescribed, rather than someone else's version or variant. What is the probability overall that the patient is correctly treated throughout?

It may be easiest to approach the problem by looking at a large throughput (say 100) of patients. With a probability of 0·9 that the consultant gets it right, thus suggests that 90 of the 100 are correctly diagnosed. Subsequently, when these 90 arrive at the clinic there is a probability of 0·7 that the treatment is exactly correct. In other words the fraction 0·7 of 90, i.e. 63 finally receive both correct diagnosis *and* correct treatment. So out of 100 people with whom we started, 63 finally get totally correct treatment. Clearly then the probability at the start that any patient gets totally correct treatment is 63/100 = 0·63, and the reader will undoubtedly have realised that we could have obtained this a little more quickly by multiplying 0·9 by 0·7. We thus have a rule:

the probability of A *and* B = probability of A times the probability of B or, in symbols,

$$P(\text{A } and \text{ B}) = P(\text{A}) \times P(\text{B})$$

(There is just one proviso: A and B need to be independent of each other.)

To take another situation, suppose that the probability that a doctor prescribes an overdose of a drug is 0·02, and that the probability a nurse fails, purely by chance, to check the dose is 0·1.

What is the probability that a patient gets an overdose? The answer is $0{\cdot}02 \times 0{\cdot}1 = 0{\cdot}002$. Putting this another way, two patients per 1000 may get an overdose.

Probability formulae

To illustrate the rules of probability let us consider the probabilities of various events connected with 100 patients, using the data in Table 43. The patients can have the correct diagnosis made, or an incorrect one. They may get the correct or incorrect treatment. It is possible that an incorrect diagnosis actually leads to the correct treatment for the real condition! (The probability of this is small.)

From the data in Table 43 we can illustrate most of the laws of probability. First, notice that since 73 out of 100 get the correct treatment

$$P(\text{correct treatment}) = 73/100$$

and since 22 get incorrect treatment

$$P(\text{incorrect treatment}) = 22/100,$$

and finally 5 are still under discussion

$$P(\text{treatment under discussion}) = 5/100$$

Talking in terms of whether treatment is correct, incorrect or under discussion, these three possibilities are *exhaustive*, i.e. include all the possibilities. The probability that the treatment is

Table 43

Cross-tabulation of Treatment and Diagnosis for 100 Patients

	Correct Diagnosis	Incorrect Diagnosis	Totals
Correct Treatment	70	3	73
Incorrect Treatment	8	14	22
Treatment under Discussion	2	3	5
Totals	80	20	100

either correct or incorrect or under discussion is 1—there are no other possibilities! Thus

$$P(\text{correct treatment } or \text{ incorrect treatment } or \text{ treatment under discussion}) = P(\text{correct treatment}) + P(\text{incorrect treatment}) + P(\text{treatment under discussion}) = 73/100 + 22/100 + 5/100 = 1$$

When a treatment is declared to be correct, this precludes it from being described as 'incorrect' or as 'under discussion'! We say that being correct, being incorrect, and being under discussion are 'mutually exclusive' states. This has implication for calculating with their probabilities. Consider, for example, the probability that a patient gets incorrect treatment *or* his treatment is still under discussion. There are 22 who get incorrect treatment, and a further separate five who are under discussion, giving 27 who fulfil one or other conditions. The probability is thus 27/100 that a patient either gets incorrect treatment *or* is still under discussion. Notice 27/100 is the sum of 22/100, the probability of incorrect treatment, and 5/100, the probability of being under discussion. Symbolically, we can write

$$P(\text{A } or \text{ B}) = P(\text{A}) + P(\text{B})$$

as long as we are dealing with mutually exclusive states or events.

Now let us consider the probability that the patient receives either a correct diagnosis, or the correct treatment (or both!). Can we add the probabilities here? If we try we get:

$$P\begin{pmatrix}\text{correct}\\\text{diagnosis}\end{pmatrix} = \frac{80}{100}$$

$$P\begin{pmatrix}\text{correct}\\\text{treatment}\end{pmatrix} = \frac{73}{100}$$

The sum of these two probabilities is 153/100. Now we know that probability has a maximum value of 1, and so clearly there is some reason why we cannot just add in this case. The reason relates to the 'mutually exclusive' idea just described. Are these two things mutually exclusive? In other words, if you get a correct diagnosis do you automatically *not* get correct treatment? Hopefully this is not the case. In fact if you get a correct diagnosis, the table strongly suggests you do get the correct treatment. What then has gone wrong? Looking back at Table 43, 80 people out of 100 had a correct diagnosis. These included, correctly, 70 who got correct treatment. When added on the 73 who got the correct treatment we included *again* the 70 who had already been counted in as having correct diagnosis. In other words simply adding the probabilities 80/100 and 73/100 has included in the 70/100 twice. The correct answer is to subtract 70/100 (who got both correct treatment *and* correct diagnosis) to avoid including them twice in the total. Thus:

$$\begin{aligned} &P(\text{correct treatment } \textit{or} \text{ correct diagnosis}) \\ &= P(\text{correct treatment}) + P(\text{correct diagnosis}) \\ &- P(\text{correct treatment } \textit{and} \text{ correct diagnosis}) \\ &= \frac{80}{100} + \frac{73}{100} - \frac{70}{100} \\ &= \frac{83}{100} \end{aligned}$$

The general rule corresponding to this is

$$P(\text{A } \textit{or} \text{ B}) = P(\text{A}) + P(\text{B}) - P(\text{A } \textit{and} \text{ B})$$

Comparing this with the 'mutually exclusive' situation above where

$$P(\text{A } \textit{or} \text{ B}) = P(\text{A}) + P(\text{B})$$

we see that the $P(\text{A } \textit{and} \text{ B})$ represents the chance of 'overlap' which, by definition, is impossible where A and B are mutually exclusive.

To illustrate the correctness of the rule, what is the probability of either incorrect treatment *or* incorrect diagnosis? We first need to decide if these events are mutually exclusive. Can we get an incorrect diagnosis *and* an incorrect treatment? The answer is yes, the events are not mutually exclusive and so we must take care with the overall probability and use

$$P(\text{A } \textit{or} \text{ B}) = P(\text{A}) + P(\text{B}) - P(\text{A } \textit{and} \text{ B})$$

where A represents 'incorrect diagnosis' and B represents 'incorrect treatment'. A *and* B represents incorrect diagnosis *and* incorrect treatment, from Table 43

$$P(\text{A}) = P(\text{incorrect diagnosis}) = \frac{20}{100}$$

$$P(\text{B}) = P(\text{incorrect treatment}) = \frac{22}{100}$$

$$P(\text{A } \textit{and} \text{ B}) = P(\text{incorrect diagnosis } \textit{and} \text{ incorrect treatment}) = \frac{14}{100}$$

hence $P(\text{A } \textit{or} \text{ B}) = P(\text{incorrect diagnosis } \textit{or} \text{ incorrect treatment})$ is

$$= \frac{20}{100} + \frac{22}{100} - \frac{14}{100}$$
$$= \frac{28}{100}$$

What is the probability that a patient who initially gets the correct diagnosis goes on later to get the correct treatment? For this we are restricting ourselves to the 80 who get the correct diagnosis, and not considering the other 20 at all. We say that we are obtaining a conditional probability. The probability is conditional that we only look at those who in the first place got the correct diagnosis. There are 80 such people, of whom, from the table we can see that 70 went on to get the correct treatment. The probability of correct treatment conditional on correct diagnosis is thus 70/80, and we write

$$P(\text{correct treatment} \mid \text{correct diagnosis}) = \frac{70}{80}$$

The $\mid$ means 'conditional on'. As another example, what is the probability of an incorrect treatment being given to someone who has had an incorrect diagnosis? There are 20 who have an incorrect diagnosis, of whom 14 then are incorrectly treated. Thus

$$P(\text{incorrect treatment} \mid \text{incorrect diagnosis}) = \frac{14}{20}$$

Notice that this is not the same as

$$P(\text{incorrect treatment } \textit{and} \text{ incorrect diagnosis})$$

From the table we are looking at the *same* 14 people, but in this latter case relating them to the 100 with whom we started, that is

$$P(\text{incorrect treatment } \textit{and} \text{ incorrect diagnosis}) = \frac{14}{100}$$

Pursuing this further how would we seek out the people who are both incorrectly diagnosed *and* incorrectly treated?

Let us start with those who are incorrectly diagnosed. There is a total of 20 of these. Moving on to the subgroup who go on to be incorrectly treated having already been incorrectly diagnosed, we see that there are 14. We have, therefore, 14 out of 100 are both incorrectly diagnosed *and* incorrectly treated. Thus

$$P(\text{incorrect diagnosis } and \text{ incorrect treatment}) = \frac{14}{100}$$

Notice the way we got at this probability. It was done in two stages. First, finding those incorrectly diagnosed, where the probability is clearly 20/100, and going on to the subset of these, namely 14/20 who also got incorrect treatment. Overall we see that a fraction, 20/100, are allowed into consideration at the first stage, and of these a fraction, 14/100, are retained as satisfying our requirements. In other words, overall 14/20 of $20/100 = 14/20 \times 20/100 = 14/100$ is the fraction who are both incorrectly diagnosed *and* incorrectly treated. This fraction is, of course, the probability obtained earlier, and we have a new approach to it by multiplying. If we put probability notation to our numbers, $20/100 = P(\text{incorrect diagnosis})$, 14/20 is $P(\text{incorrect treatment} \mid \text{incorrect diagnosis})$ and 14/100 is $P(\text{incorrect diagnosis } and \text{ incorrect treatment})$. The law which then emerges is:

$$\begin{aligned} &P(\text{incorrect treatment } and \text{ incorrect diagnosis}) \\ &= P(\text{incorrect diagnosis}) \times P(\text{incorrect treatment} \mid \text{incorrect diagnosis}) \end{aligned}$$

In symbols, if A represents incorrect diagnosis, and B represents incorrect treatment, then

$$P(\text{A } and \text{ B}) = P(\text{A}) \times P(\text{B} \mid \text{A})$$

This is the multiplication law of probability. As an example, suppose that 60% of sufferers from coronary thrombosis survive the first 24 hours. Of those who are thus fortunate, suppose 25% survive 10 years. In probability terms

$$P(\text{patient survives 24 hours}) = 0{\cdot}6$$
$$P(\text{patient survives 10 years} \mid \text{he survives 24 hours}) = 0{\cdot}25$$

Therefore

$$\begin{aligned} &P(\text{patient survives 10 years}) \\ &= P(\text{patient survives 24 hours}) \times P(\text{patient survives 10 years} \mid \text{he survives 24 hours}) \\ &= 0{\cdot}6 \times 0{\cdot}25 \\ &= 0{\cdot}15 \end{aligned}$$

Earlier on in this section we had a similar formula:

$$P(\text{A } \textit{and} \text{ B}) = P(\text{A}) \times (\text{B})$$

with the proviso that A and B were independent. This earlier rule is then a special case of the more general rule now obtained. Looking at the general multiplication rule, if $P(\text{B} \mid \text{A})$ is the same as $P(\text{B})$, this implies that B is not conditional on A but is independent. Take for example the probability of scores 2 *and* 3 in two tosses of a die. According to the general multiplication rule:

$$P(2 \textit{ and } 3) = P(2) \times P(3 \mid 2)$$

Now $P(2) = 1/6$ assuming the die is fair and $P(3 \mid 2)$ is also 1/6, and is the same as $P(3)$. Whether we get a 3 on our second toss is quite independent of what happened on our first toss. The solution then can be written more simply as

$$P(2 \textit{ and } 3) = P(2) \times P(3)$$

using our earlier multiplication law for independent events.

Let us return now to reconsidering P(incorrect diagnosis *and* incorrect treatment), and try it another way. We could look at those patients who got incorrect treatment, and trace them back to see if they were incorrectly diagnosed, thus reversing our search procedure. Twenty-two patients were incorrectly treated and, from Table 43, 14 of these were incorrectly diagnosed. We have of course reached the same 14 as before. The steps in the calculation are, firstly, to say that there is proportion 22/100 who get incorrect treatment, and of these the fraction 14/22 had incorrect diagnosis. Thus, overall a proportion $22/100 \times 14/22 = 14/100$ received both incorrect diagnosis and incorrect treatment. As before we have a multiplication process which in probability terms looks like this:

$$P(\text{incorrect treatment}) \times P(\text{incorrect diagnosis} \mid \text{incorrect treatment})$$
$$= P(\text{incorrect treatment } \textit{and} \text{ incorrect diagnosis})$$

Going back to our symbols where A represents incorrect diagnosis and B represents incorrect treatment, we have $P(\text{B}) \times P(\text{A} \mid \text{B}) = P(\text{B } \textit{and} \text{ A})$. We can also note that $P(\text{B } \textit{and} \text{ A})$ is the same as $P(\text{A } \textit{and} \text{ B})$, or put another way, incorrect treatment and incorrect diagnosis is the same as incorrect diagnosis and incorrect treatment.

We can now collect together our two alternative formulae for multiplication:

$$P(\text{A } and \text{ B}) = P(\text{A}) \times P(\text{B} \mid \text{A}) = P(\text{B}) \times P(\text{A} \mid \text{B})$$

More Complicated Formulations

For some applications we use only the second and third parts of this expression. Thus

$$P(\text{A}) \times P(\text{B} \mid \text{A}) = P(\text{B}) \times P(\text{A} \mid \text{B})$$

For example, if we divide both sides by $P(\text{B})$, we obtain

$$\frac{P(\text{A}) \times P(\text{B} \mid \text{A})}{P(\text{B})} = P(\text{A} \mid \text{B})$$

Suppose we know prior to our analysis that $P(\text{B}) = P(\text{incorrect treatment}) = 22/100$, that $P(\text{A}) = P(\text{incorrect diagnosis}) = 20/100$ and that $P(\text{B} \mid \text{A}) = P(\text{incorrect treatment} \mid \text{incorrect diagnosis}) = 14/20$. We can then derive $P(\text{A} \mid \text{B})$, which is the probability that an incorrect diagnosis was made in the first place, given that we now observe an incorrect treatment being given:

$$P(\text{A}|\text{B}) = \frac{\frac{20}{100} \times \frac{14}{20}}{\frac{22}{100}}$$

$$= \frac{\cancel{20}}{\cancel{100}} \times \frac{14}{\cancel{20}} \times \frac{\cancel{100}}{22}$$

$$= \frac{14}{22}$$

This rather peculiar probability should be regarded as an updated version of $P(\text{A})$, the probability of incorrect diagnosis.†

† *Footnote on Subjective Probability:* There is here something of a philosophical difficulty which causes argument among statisticians. Probability, according to some statisticians, is a measure applied to a future situation. In the case we are considering, the events have already happened and so some would argue that this part of our exercise is not valid or needed. There are, however, useful spin-offs to be obtained by allowing our definition of probability as 'the legitimate intensity of belief' to prevail. We can then say: how intensely do we believe that a patient who has the incorrect treatment was also previously subjected to the incorrect

We knew in advance that $P(\text{A})$ was 20/100. After observing incorrect treatment we have modified or 'revised' $P(\text{A})$ to a new value $P(\text{A} \mid \text{B})$, which is 14/22. The new information that incorrect treatment has been observed has caused revision of the 'prior' probability $P(\text{A})$ of 20/100 to the 'posterior' probability $P(\text{A} \mid \text{B})$ of 14/22, making it appear more likely now than previously that a wrong diagnosis was made. The expression

$$P(\text{A} \mid \text{B}) = \frac{P(\text{A}) \times P(\text{B} \mid \text{A})}{P(\text{B})}$$

is known as Bayes' rule, and in the following sections we develop an expanded version which, whilst looking somewhat more complicated, is conceptually nothing more than the above expression.

Let us consider three possible mutually exclusive diagnoses A_1, A_2 and A_3 and an observed symptom B in a patient. From experience suppose we know that when illness A_1 is present there is a probability that symptom B occurs. Thus, $P(\text{B} \mid \text{A}_1) = 0{\cdot}4$. We also know that when A_2 is present we might get B with a probability 0·2. Thus, $P(\text{B} \mid \text{A}_2) = 0{\cdot}2$. And, finally, we might get B as a result of A_3 with a probability 0·1 thus $P(\text{B} \mid \text{A}_3) = 0{\cdot}1$. We also know that the list A_1, A_2 and A_3 is exhaustive. That is, B definitely results from one of A_1 or A_2 or A_3. We now seek the probability of observing symptom B in a patient. This comes from the probability that A_1 occurs *and* then B follows, *or* the probability that A_2 occurs *and* then B follows, *or* the probability A_3 occurs *and* then B follows. The three parts of this probability each separated by '*or*' contribute to the total, and as they are mutually exclusive we can invoke the addition rule† to add them thus:

$$P(\text{B}) = P(\text{A}_1 \textit{ and } \text{then B}) + P(\text{A}_2 \textit{ and } \text{then B}) + P(\text{A}_3 \textit{ and } \text{then B})$$

notice that each '*or*' becomes a plus sign. Looking at the three terms on the right hand side, we see that each is amenable to application of the multiplication rule obtained earlier. Thus, as an example,

$$P(\text{A}_1 \textit{ and } \text{then B}) = P(\text{A}_1) \times P(\text{B} \mid \text{A}_1)$$

diagnosis. It is true that it has happened and *is* or *is not* establishable fact. But it is also true that we may not have any way of establishing the truth, and need to make a probability calculation appertaining to likelihood of the various possibilities that might have occurred.

† What we have intuitively done is to extend the mutually exclusive addition rule $P(\text{A } \textit{or} \text{ B}) = P(\text{A}) + P(\text{B})$ given earlier to $P(\text{A } \textit{or} \text{ B } \textit{or} \text{ C}) = P(\text{A}) + P(\text{B}) + P(\text{C})$.

Putting this into the expression for $P(\mathrm{B})$, together with the comparable versions for (A_2 *and* then B) and (A_3 *and* then B) we obtain:

$$P(\mathrm{B}) = P(\mathrm{A}_1) \times P(\mathrm{B} \mid \mathrm{A}_1) + P(\mathrm{A}_2) \times P(\mathrm{B} \mid \mathrm{A}_2) + P(\mathrm{A}_3) \times P(\mathrm{B} \mid \mathrm{A}_3)$$

This is the *rule of elimination*, and it says that the probability we observe B is made up of various parts, dependent on the alternative sources of B.

At this point it is opportune to take another look at Bayes' rule given earlier. If we replace the A by A_1 in the rule we obtain

$$P(\mathrm{A}_1 \mid \mathrm{B}) = \frac{P(\mathrm{A}_1) \times P(\mathrm{B} \mid \mathrm{A}_1)}{P(\mathrm{B})}$$

Now we know that there are three possible diagnoses A_1, A_2 and A_3 which can cause B. When we seek $P(\mathrm{A}_1 \mid \mathrm{B})$ we are revising a prior notion of $P(\mathrm{A}_1)$ in the light of having observed B in a patient.

To obtain $P(\mathrm{B})$, the denominator in Bayes' rule, we use the rule of elimination above:

$$P(\mathrm{B}) = P(\mathrm{A}_1) \times P(\mathrm{B} \mid \mathrm{A}_1) + P(\mathrm{A}_2) \times P(\mathrm{B} \mid \mathrm{A}_2) + P(\mathrm{A}_3) \times P(\mathrm{B} \mid \mathrm{A}_3)$$

Substituting this rule into the denominator we obtain

$$P(\mathrm{A}_1 \mid \mathrm{B}) = \frac{P(\mathrm{A}_1) \times P(\mathrm{B} \mid \mathrm{A}_1)}{P(\mathrm{A}_1) \times P(\mathrm{B} \mid \mathrm{A}_1) + P(\mathrm{A}_2) \times P(\mathrm{B} \mid \mathrm{A}_2) + P(\mathrm{A}_3) \times P(\mathrm{B} \mid \mathrm{A}_3)}$$

which is the full formula for Bayes' rule.

If there were more than three possible diagnoses then the denominator on the right hand side would be expanded accordingly to include them. The formulae for $P(\mathrm{A}_2 \mid \mathrm{B})$ and $P(\mathrm{A}_3 \mid \mathrm{B})$ are obtained by altering A_1 to A_2 or A_3 as appropriate on the left hand side and in the numerator of the right hand side.

We stated earlier that $P(\mathrm{B} \mid \mathrm{A}_1) = 0{\cdot}4$, $P(\mathrm{B} \mid \mathrm{A}_2) = 0{\cdot}2$ and $P(\mathrm{B} \mid \mathrm{A}_3) = 0{\cdot}1$. Suppose also we know that in the population being considered, the incidence in general of A_1 is 20 per thousand, of A_2 is 30 per thousand and of A_3 is 40 per thousand. Remembering that A_1, A_2 and A_3 are mutually exclusive, we have $20 + 30 + 40 = 90$ cases per 1000 of the illnesses in question. So we know in advance that if 90 people are recorded ill, then the proportion having A_1 is 20/90, i.e. $P(\mathrm{A}_1) = 20/90 = 0{\cdot}222$ and $P(\mathrm{A}_2) = 30/90 = 0{\cdot}333$ and $P(\mathrm{A}_3) = 40/90 = 0{\cdot}444$. From Bayes' rule, after observing symptom B in a patient, we revise $P(\mathrm{A}_1)$ from 0·222 to $P(\mathrm{A}_1 \mid \mathrm{B})$ which is:

$$\frac{0{\cdot}02 \times 0{\cdot}4}{0{\cdot}02 \times 0{\cdot}4 + 0{\cdot}03 \times 0{\cdot}2 + 0{\cdot}04 \times 0{\cdot}1} = 0{\cdot}444$$

We thus in this case have doubled the prior probability $P(A_1)$ to obtain the posterior probability $P(A_1 \mid B)$.

This idea of revising probability ties in with remarks made in both the introduction to this book, and the introduction to this chapter. Recall that prior to a surgical operation we speculated that the probability of success was 0·5, or 50%, but that as some progress was made, and thus as new information came to light, the probability was subjectively revised to 0·6, or 60%. Bayes' rule is the formal equivalent of this revision.

Probability Distributions

Empirical versus theoretical histograms

The histogram shown in Fig. 8(a) represents a picture of the density of the data around the mean. The *actual* frequencies are shown by the areas of the blocks. An alternative perspective was (Fig. 8(b)) to consider the areas as showing the *relative frequency* of occurrence of the various classes. Thus, class 1 to 1·1 occurs six times or, in relative frequency terms, 6/70 or 8·6% of the time. No alteration is required to the diagram, but the scale has to be read in per cent since the areas now represent percentages or fractions. Clearly, the total area under the histogram is 100% or 1. If we were to select a birthweight at random we would say there is a probability of 6/70 that it will fall in the range 1 to 1·1. 'Relative frequency' as we have said, provides the basic concept of probability. Thus, the probability that a randomly chosen baby will exceed 1·40 kg would be the percentage, i.e. the area to the right of 140, i.e. 40% or 0·40.

Inference and hypothesis testing and other applications of statistics are built up from histograms, sometimes obtained empirically as with the birthweights, but frequently obtained theoretically. A number of well-documented shapes of histograms occur regularly among which the Binomial, Poisson and normal distributions are the most common and useful. These theoretical relative frequency histograms are known as 'probability distributions'.

The Binomial distribution

Suppose we looked at a family of six children and said: how many boys might there be? There are obviously seven possibilities: any number from 0 to 6 inclusive. If we could work out a probability for each of the numbers 0 to 6 inclusive and put these into a table, then we would have a probability distribution. We could then draw a diagram rather like a histogram showing the various probabilities.

There is something quite distinctive about the probability distribution for the number of boys or girls in a family. In such a situation there are only two outcomes—boy or girl—and we assume that the probability of a boy does not change throughout, however many boys or girls are born. The probability is thus constant, and each event, i.e. the sex of each new baby, is independent of its predecessor. When these assumptions are met, we can find the probabilities of the various possible outcomes by the use of the Binomial formula. A similar situation could occur when a patient on a life support system in an intensive care unit has three separate indicators, any of which would indicate some sort of equipment failure. If a failure occurs any one or any two or all three indicators might function. Or none may function. The outcomes 'function' or 'not function' are like the outcomes 'boy' or 'girl'. Just as we assumed that there was a constant probability of a boy, so now we would need to assume that each of the indicators had the same chance of working. And, as we assumed that a history of, for example, boys did not alter the probability of a subsequent boy, so we now assume that the fact that say two indicators function has no effect whatsoever on the chance that the other works.

The calculation of Binomial probabilities is routine, either by the formula or by reading them from a table. All we need to know is the number, n, of 'trials' (e.g. children in the family), and the probability, p, of the particular outcome of interest (e.g. a boy).

Of perhaps more interest is an extreme case of the Binomial distribution in which the number of trials is very large, and the probability of an outcome is very small. The incidence of a rare disease in a population is such an example. Suppose that in a population of 50 000 000 people there is a probability of 1/5 000 000 of contracting in a year, legionnaire's disease. This would suggest that on average we might get ten new cases per year ($50\,000\,000 \times 1/5\,000\,000$).

It is reasonable to assume that the Binomial conditions (described earlier) are met here†, and so in theory any probability can be worked out. The Binomial tables don't cover such a large number of trials (50 000 000), and the calculations involved, because of the magnitudes of the numbers, are tedious, especially if we require, for example, a combined probability, such as the probability of 15 to 20 cases per year. In this situation, where we deal with a very large number of trials (i.e. people) and a very small probability, we use a much simpler formula known as the Poisson distribution formula. Another example might be the number of cardiac infarctions in a day in a city of 1 million people. The number of trials (i.e. people) is large, and the probability of onset of cardiac infarction is small, for any person, and might provide on average a handful of cases. When planning facilities for the care of such cases, the Poisson probability formula can play an important role.

The normal distribution

The other related distribution is the normal, a bell shape which occurs with amazing regularity. It is perhaps best known because it occurs with IQs, usually normally distributed around a mean of 100. The normal distribution is a close relative of the Binomial distribution and provides a further good alternative for use in computing Binomial probabilities when the Binomial formula is too tedious to use. The normal distribution is of fundamental importance in sampling theory and is discussed in Chapters 4 and 5. All three of these 'theoretical' distributions, together with others, permit the statistician to understand the randomness and variability in processes without the need to take specific measures and collect expensive data.

Some Formulae

The Binomial distribution

n = number of trials.
$n! = n \times (n-1) \times (n-2) \times \ldots \times 2 \times 1$
(pronounced 'n factorial').

The Poisson distribution

Notation as for Binomial distribution.

† The independence condition may be violated if we accept that people get the disease in groups, perhaps from staying at the same hotel. We will ignore this possibility here.

$r! = r(r-1) \times (r-2) \times (r-3) \ldots \times 1$.
$(n-r)! = (n-r) \times (n-r-1) \times (n-r-2) \times (n-r-3) \times \ldots \times 1$
p = probability that the outcome occurs at any trial.
$P(r)$ = the probability that in n trials there are r of the particular outcome.

$$P(r) = \frac{n!}{r!\,(n-r)!}\,p^r(1-p)^{n-r}.$$

The mean number of successes is $n \times p$. The standard deviation of the number of successes is $\sqrt{n \times p \times (1-p)}$.

The mean $= n \times p$. The standard deviation is $\sqrt{n \times p}$.
$e = 2{\cdot}718\ldots$

$$P(r) = \frac{(\text{mean})^r\,e^{-\text{mean}}}{r!}.$$

Appendix 3: Statistical Tables

Table in Appendix 3a was taken from;

Robert D. Mason, *Essentials of Statistics*, Prentice-Hall, Inc., 1976.

Table in Appendix 3b was taken from:

Table III of Fisher and Yates, *Statistical Tables for Biological, Agricultural and Medical Research*, published by Longman Group Ltd., London (previously published by Oliver & Boyd, Edinburgh) and by permission of the authors and publishers.

Table in Appendix 3d was taken from:

W.J. Conover, *Practical Nonparametric Statistics*, John Wiley & Sons, Inc., New York, 1971.

Appendix 3a: Areas under the standard normal probability distribution between the mean and successive values of *z*

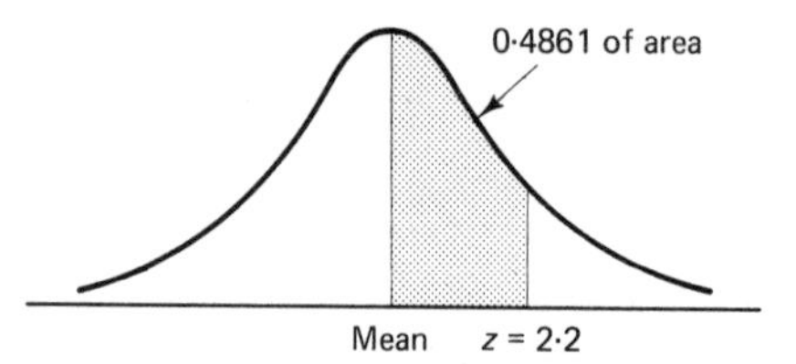

Example: To find the area under the curve between the mean and a point 2·2 standard deviations to the right of the mean, look up the value opposite 2·2 in the table; 0·4861 of the area under the curve lies between the mean and a *z* value of 2·2.

z	00	.01	.02	.03	.04	.05	.06	.07	.08	.09
0.0	.0000	.0040	.0080	.0120	.0160	.0199	.0239	.0279	.0319	.0359
0.1	.0398	.0438	.0478	.0517	.0557	.0596	.0636	.0675	.0714	.0753
0.2	.0793	.0832	.0871	.0910	.0948	.0987	.1026	.1064	.1103	.1141
0.3	.1179	.1217	.1255	.1293	.1331	.1368	.1406	.1443	.1480	.1517
0.4	.1554	.1591	.1628	.1664	.1700	.1736	.1772	.1808	.1844	.1879
0·5	.1915	·1950	.1985	.2019	.2054	.2088	.2123	.2157	.2190	.2224
0.6	.2257	.2291	.2324	.2357	.2389	.2422	.2454	.2486	.2517	.2549
0.7	.2580	.2611	.2642	.2673	.2704	.2734	.2764	.2794	.2823	.2852
0·8	.2881	.2910	.2939	.2967	.2995	.3023	.3051	.3078	.3106	.3133
0.9	.3159	.3186	.3212	.3238	.3264	.3289	.3315	.3340	.3365	.3389
1.0	.3413	.3438	.3461	.3485	.3508	.3531	.3554	.3577	.3599	.3621
1.1	.3643	.3665	.3686	.3708	.3729	.3749	.3770	.3790	.3810	.3830
1.2	.3849	.3869	.3888	.3907	.3925	.3944	.3962	.3980	.3997	.4015
1.3	.4032	.4049	.4066	.4082	.4099	.4115	.4131	.4147	.4162	.4177
1.4	.4192	.4207	.4222	.4236	.4251	.4265	.4279	.4292	.4306	.4319
1.5	.4332	.4345	.4357	.4370	.4382	.4394	.4406	.4418	.4429	.4441
1.6	.4452	.4463	.4474	.4484	.4495	.4505	.4515	.4525	.4535	.4545
1.7	.4554	.4564	.4573	.4582	.4591	.4599	.4608	.4616	.4625	.4633
1.8	.4641	.4649	.4656	.4664	.4671	.4678	.4686	.4693	.4699	.4706
1.9	.4713	.4719	.4726	.4732	.4738	.4744	.4750	.4756	.4761	.4767
2.0	.4772	.4778	.4783	.4788	.4793	.4798	.4803	.4808	.4812	.4817
2.1	.4821	.4826	.4830	.4834	.4838	.4842	.4846	.4850	.4854	.4857
2.2	.4861	.4864	.4868	.4871	.4875	.4878	.4881	.4884	.4887	.4890
2.3	.4893	.4896	.4898	.4901	.4904	.4906	.4909	.4911	.4913	.4916
2.4	.4918	.4920	.4922	.4925	.4927	.4929	.4931	.4932	.4934	.4936
2.5	.4938	.4940	.4941	.4943	.4945	.4946	.4948	.4949	.4951	.4952
2.6	.4953	.4955	.4956	.4957	.4959	.4960	.4961	.4962	.4963	.4946
2.7	.4965	.4966	.4967	.4968	.4969	.4970	.4971	.4972	.4973	.4974
2.8	.4974	.4975	.4976	.4977	.4977	.4978	.4979	.4979	.4980	.4981
2.9	.4981	.4982	.4982	.4983	.4984	.4984	.4985	.4985	.4986	.4986
3.0	.4987	.4987	.4987	.4988	.4988	.4989	.4989	.4989	.4990	.4990

Appendix 3b: Areas in both tails combined for Student's *t* distribution

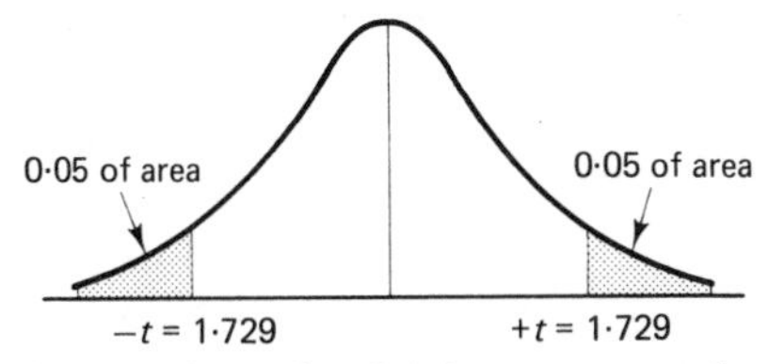

Example: To find the value of *t* which corresponds to an area of 0·10 in both tails of the distribution combined, when there are 19 degrees of freedom, look under the 0·10 column, and proceed down to the 19 degrees of freedom row; the appropriate *t* value there is 1·729.

Degrees of Freedom	Area in Both Tails Combined .10	.05	.02	.01
1	6.314	12.706	31.821	63.657
2	2.920	4.303	6.965	9.925
3	2.353	3.182	4.541	5.841
4	2.132	2.776	3.747	4.604
5	2.015	2.571	3.365	4.032
6	1.943	2.447	3.143	3.707
7	1.895	2.365	2.998	3.499
8	1.860	2.306	2.896	3.355
9	1.833	2.262	2.821	3.250
10	1.812	2.228	2.764	3.169
11	1.796	2.201	2.718	3.106
12	1.782	2.179	2.681	3.055
13	1.771	2.160	2.650	3.012
14	1.761	2.145	2.624	2.977
15	1.753	2.131	2.602	2.947
16	1.746	2.120	2.583	2.921
17	1.740	2.110	2.567	2.898
18	1.734	2.101	2.552	2.878
19	1.729	2.093	2.539	2.861
20	1.725	2.086	2.528	2.845
21	1.721	2.080	2.518	2.831
22	1.717	2.074	2.508	2.819
23	1.714	2.069	2.500	2.807
24	1.711	2.064	2.492	2.797
25	1.708	2.060	2.485	2.787
26	1.706	2.056	2.479	2.779
27	1.703	2.052	2.473	2.771
28	1.701	2.048	2.467	2.763
29	1.699	2.045	2.462	2.756
30	1.697	2.042	2.457	2.750
40	1.684	2.021	2.423	2.704
60	1.671	2.000	2.390	2.660
120	1.658	1.980	2.358	2.617
Normal distribution	1.645	1.960	2.326	2.576

Appendix 3c: Area in the right tail of a chi-square distribution

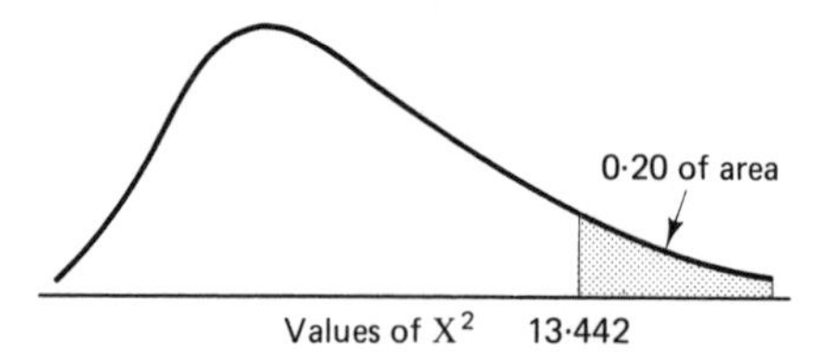

Example: In a chi-square distribution with 10 degrees of freedom, if we want to find the appropriate chi-square value for 0·20 of the area under the curve (the shaded area in the right tail) we look under the 0·20 column in the table and proceed down to the 10 degrees of freedom row; the appropriate chi-square value there is 13·442.

Area in Right Tail					Degrees of Freedom
.20	.10	.05	.025	.01	
1.642	2.706	3.841	5.024	6.635	1
3.219	4.605	5.991	7.378	9.210	2
4.642	6.251	7.815	9.348	11.345	3
5.989	7.779	9.488	11.143	13.277	4
7.289	9.236	11.070	12.833	15.086	5
8.558	10.645	12.592	14.449	16.812	6
9.803	12.017	14.067	16.013	18.475	7
11.030	13.362	15.507	17.535	20.090	8
12.242	14.684	16.919	19.023	21.666	9
13.442	15.987	18.307	20.483	23.209	10
14.631	17.275	19.675	21.920	24.725	11
15.812	18.549	21.026	23.337	26.217	12
16.985	19.812	22.362	24.736	27.688	13
18.151	21.064	23.685	26.119	29.141	14
19.311	22.307	24.996	27.488	30.578	15
20.465	23.542	26.296	28.845	32.000	16
21.615	24.769	27.587	30.191	33.409	17
22.760	25.989	28.869	31.526	34.805	18
23.900	27.204	30.144	32.852	36.191	19
25.038	28.412	31.410	34.170	37.566	20
26.171	29.615	32.671	35.479	38.932	21
27.301	30.813	33.924	36.781	40.289	22
28.429	32.007	35.172	38.076	41.638	23
29.553	33.196	36.415	39.364	42.980	24
30.675	34.382	37.652	40.647	44.314	25
31.795	35.563	38.885	41.923	45.642	26
32.912	36.741	40.113	43.194	46.963	27
34.027	37.916	41.337	44.461	48.278	28
35.139	39.087	42.557	45.722	49.588	29
36.250	40.256	43.773	46.979	50.892	30

Appendix 3d: Values for Spearman's rank correlation (r_s) for combined areas in both tails

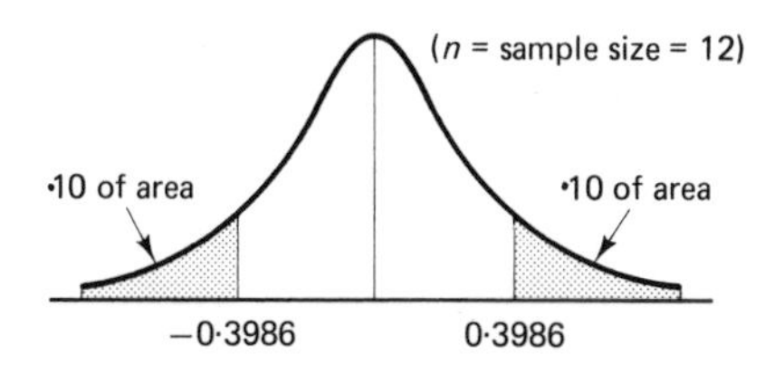

Example: For a two-tailed test of significance at the 0·20 level, with $n = 12$, the appropriate value for r_s can be found by looking under the 0·20 column and proceeding down to the 12 row; there we find the appropriate r_s value to be 0·3986.

n	.20	.10	.05	.02	.01	.002
4	.8000	.8000				
5	.7000	.8000	.9000	.9000		
6	.6000	.7714	.8286	.8857	.9429	
7	.5357	.6786	.7450	.8571	.8929	.9643
8	.5000	.6190	.7143	.8095	.8571	.9286
9	.4667	.5833	.6833	.7667	.8167	.9000
10	.4424	.5515	.6364	.7333	.7818	.8667
11	.4182	.5273	.6091	.7000	.7455	.8364
12	.3986	.4965	.5804	.6713	.7273	.8182
13	.3791	.4780	.5549	.6429	.6978	.7912
14	.3626	.4593	.5341	.6220	.6747	.7670
15	.3500	.4429	.5179	.6000	.6536	.7464
16	.3382	.4265	.5000	.5824	.6324	.7265
17	.3260	.4118	.4853	.5637	.6152	.7083
18	.3148	.3994	.4716	.5480	.5975	.6904
19	.3070	.3895	.4579	.5333	.5825	.6737
20	.2977	.3789	.4451	.5203	.5684	.6586
21	.2909	.3688	.4351	.5078	.5545	.6455
22	.2829	.3597	.4241	.4963	.5426	.6318
23	.2767	.3518	.4150	.4852	.5306	.6186
24	.2704	.3435	.4061	.4748	.5200	.6070
25	.2646	.3362	.3977	.4654	.5100	.5962
26	.2588	.3299	.3894	.4564	.5002	.5856
27	.2540	.3236	.3822	.4481	.4915	.5757
28	.2490	.3175	.3749	.4401	.4828	.5660
29	.2443	.3113	.3685	.4320	.4744	.5567
30	.2400	.3059	.3620	.4251	.4665	.5479

Appendix 3d: Contd.

Examples to illustrate the use of the table for rank correlation

(1) For a two-tailed test of association at the 5% level with ten pairs of observations, the rank correlation obtained must exceed 0·6364 to be able to reject the null hypothesis of no association. The two-tailed test is used where there are no grounds for deciding whether the rank correlation should be positive or negative.

(2) For a one-tailed test of association at the 5% level with ten pairs of observations, the rank correlation obtained must exceed 0·5515 to reject the null hypothesis of no association. The one-tailed test is used where there are clear grounds for expecting a positive (or negative) rank correlation.

Appendix 3e: Test values to be exceeded for the coefficient of simple correlation to be significant

Number of Points on Scatter Graph	10% Significance Level	5% Significance Level	1% Significance Level
3	0.988	0.997	1.00
4	0.900	0.950	0.99
5	0.805	0.878	0.95
6	0.729	0.811	0.91
7	0.669	0.755	0.87
8	0.621	0.707	0.83
9	0.582	0.666	0.79
10	0.549	0.632	0.76
11	0.521	0.602	0.73
12	0.497	0.576	0.70
13	0.476	0.553	0.68
14	0.457	0.532	0.66
15	0.441	0.514	0.64
16	0.426	0.497	0.62
17	0.412	0.482	0.60
18	0.400	0.468	0.59
19	0.389	0.456	0.57
20	0.378	0.444	0.56
21	0.369	0.433	0.54
22	0.360	0.423	0.53
23	0.352	0.413	0.52
24	0.344	0.406	0.51
25	0.337	0·396	0·50
26	0.330	0.388	0.49
27	0.323	0.381	0.48
28	0.317	0.374	0.47
29	0.311	0.367	0.47
30	0.306	0.361	0.46
35	0.283	0.335	0.43
40	0.264	0.312	0.40
45	0.249	0.294	0.38
50	0.235	0.279	0.36
60	0.215	0.255	0.33
70	0.198	0.236	0.30
80	0.185	0.220	0.28
90	0.175	0.207	0.27

Index

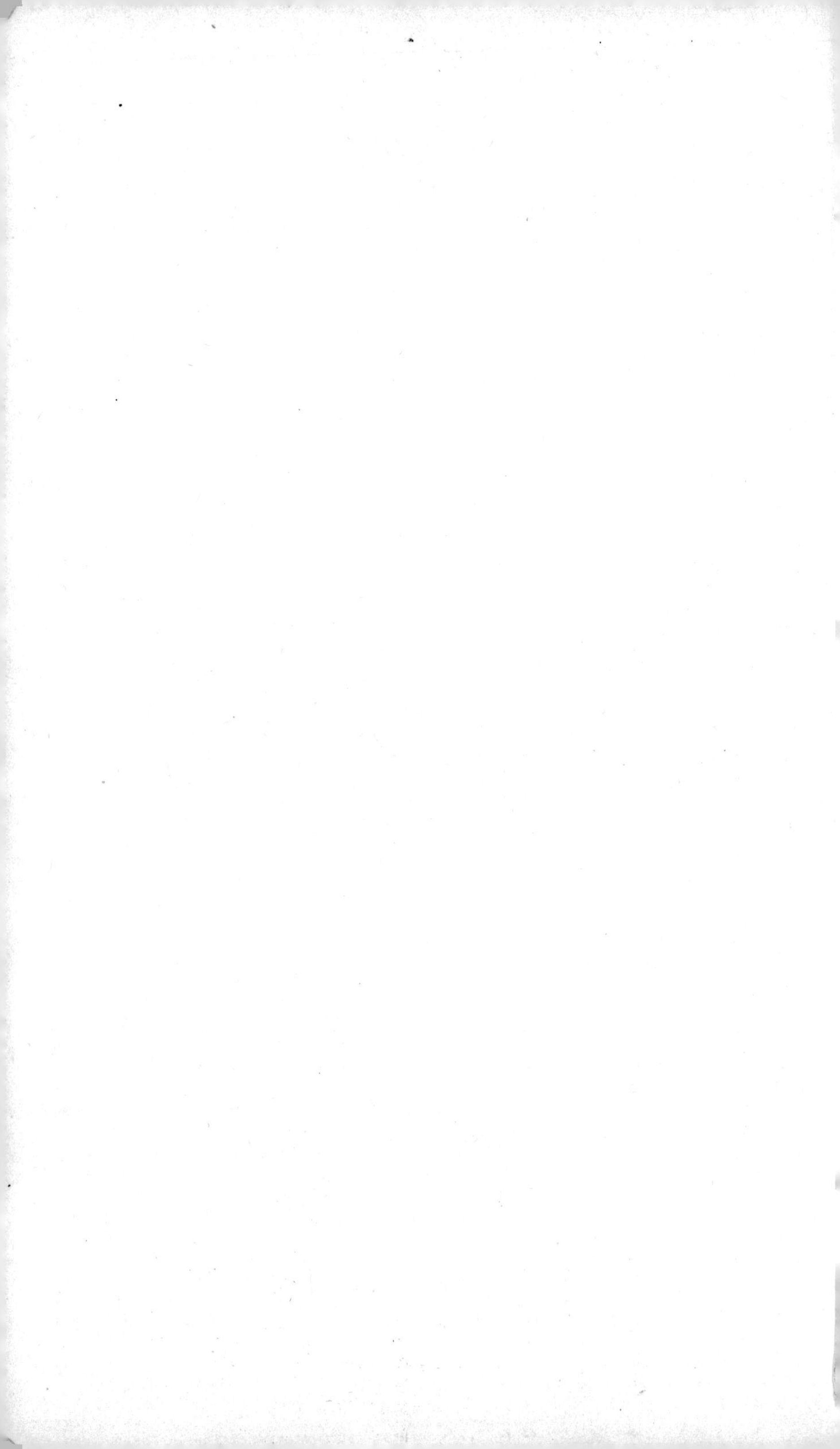